Leadership in Unconventional Crises

A Transatlantic and Cross-Sector Assessment

By

Erwan Lagadec

Lagadec, Erwan, *Leadership in Unconventional Crises, A Transatlantic and Cross-Sector Assessment* (Washington, D.C.: Center for Transatlantic Relations, 2009).

Center for Transatlantic Relations
The Paul H. Nitze School of Advanced International Studies
The Johns Hopkins University
1717 Massachusetts Ave., NW, Suite 525
Washington, D.C. 20036
Tel. (202) 663-5880
Fax (202) 663-5879
Email: transatlantic@jhu.edu
http://transatlantic.sais-jhu.edu

ISBN 13: 978-0-9841341-0-6

Cover picture: Albrecht Altdorfer (1480-1538), "The Battle of Issus" (detail), image courtesy of Bayerische Staatsgemäldesammlungen—Alte Pinakothek Munich.

Table of Contents

Acknowledgments ix

Introduction 1

The Certainty of the Unthinkable 11

Asking the Right Questions 19

    What is the essence of the crisis? 21

        The danger of premature labels 21

        Labeling crises down 21

        The illusion of self-evident characterizations 22

        Against technical categorizations: the human dimension 28

        Categorizing oneself 30

    What are the critical pitfalls? 31

        Groupthink and conventional paradigms 31

        Lethal unintended consequences 33

        Self-defeating plans 34

        Loss of trust 37

        Mismanaging imperfect information 42

        Leaving ethical questions unresolved 43

        Ready-made thought processes 45

        The artificial reassertion of normalcy: fighting the last war . . . 45

        Failures of imagination: the illusion of relevance 47

        Stovepipes and blind spots in partnerships 50

    Who are the unconventional stakeholders? 51

        The few and the many 52

        Differentiation of relevance 57

What initiatives can be taken to recover traction
on events? 59

   Creating unconventional coalitions 60

   Recovering control over the pace of crisis 67

Unconventional Crisis Cells 69

Overview of mechanisms and concepts 69

   Electricité de France: Rapid Reflection Force 69

   Afghanistan: "intellectual swarming" 77

   Mapping networks: "hubmasters" and "hubwatch" 78

The case for "horizon-scanning" and "red teams":
unconventional training exercise 79

   The essence of the crisis 80

   Critical pitfalls 82

   Mapping partners and spoilers 85

   Critical initiatives 87

Redrawing Cross-Sector Allocations of Tasks 91

Public sector perspectives 91

   Building cross-sector fields of vision 91

   Cross-silo response efforts 93

   Preventing "orphan crises" 95

Views from other sectors 96

   Calling on government to do its job 96

   Understanding the private sector 97

   The irrelevance of public sector suspicion 98

   New social compact vs. government withdrawal 98

Enhancing Systemic Resiliency 101

Structural resiliency 101

Superstructure resiliency 102

Lifeblood resiliency: the human dimension 104

Distributed leadership 106
The resiliency of narratives 107

The "Alignment" of International Responders 109

Coordination mechanisms 110
The EU platform 110
The UN platform 110
From unity of command to unity of effort 113
Structure and culture of mutual aid 115

Alignment 115
Core culture and coalescence 115
Incentive structures: leverage and narrative 117
Pervasive information 118
Enhancing local capacity: bottom-up alignment 120

Education, Training, and the Culture of Leaders . . . 123

The problem with leadership culture 123
Unconventional training 128
Unconventional leadership skills 134
Towards new criteria for the selection of leaders 139
Group dynamics 141

Conclusion 143

Annex I: Interviews 147

Annex II: Participants 155

Annex III: Seminar Program, April 10-11, 2008 157

Annex IV: Contents of 2008 Report 161

About the Author 162

About the Center 163

We are like sorcerers' apprentices, overwhelmed by complexity that we created ourselves.

Nous sommes les apprentis sorciers d'une complexité dont nous sommes les propres auteurs.

—*A participant in our 2008 seminar*

Acknowledgments

In the opening paragraph of the 2008 report where I laid out the initial results of the *Unconventional Crises* project, I expressed my gratitude to friends and colleagues who had taken the first "leap in the dark" with me, as we embarked on a project that aimed to be as unconventional as the events it examined.

Building upon these early dynamics to bring our efforts to maturity turned out to be an equally daunting proposition, though the nature of the obstacles may have changed. The experience has been all the more rewarding as we met the challenge through a collective effort, which brought old friends and new partners together.

At the intersection between the worlds of academia and policy-making, the Center for Transatlantic Relations at Johns Hopkins University's School of Advanced International Studies has remained the ideal home to build a transnational platform for analysis and action among different sectors, aiming to influence both decision-making and educational efforts with intellectual independence, rigor, and audacity. My thanks go to the Center's directors Drs. Dan Hamilton, and, especially, Esther Brimmer.

Our colleague Mike Granatt often quotes a line from Shakespeare's *Henry VIII* which suggests that leaders' "evil manners live in brass; their virtues we write in water." That is true, of course: except that good leaders, once they move on, will make their virtues spectacularly evident to those they leave behind. Esther's departure to the State Department has left just such an eloquent vacuum, whose impact cannot be fully mitigated by the recognition that such transitions are in the nature of Washington think tanks; that she will do a magnificent job in her new responsibilities; and that a much broader audience will now have a chance to write her virtues in brass.

Just as he had decisively contributed to lift our project off the ground, Pierre Béroux, *Directeur du Contrôle des Risques* at Electricité de France, has remained its driving force over the past year through his continued financial, but also intellectual support. On the American side, J. Michael Hickey at Verizon played an equally critical part in ensuring that our project gained added momentum, and in shaping its objectives as it did. One of the perks of turning a pilot project into a longer-term endeavor has been to see colleagues become sponsors—and sponsors become friends: our thanks go to Janice Maragakis from Accor North America; Nan Buzard from the American Red Cross; François-Xavier Desjars and Robert Noonan from Société Générale. We also appreciate the generous support of the Paris-based French American Foundation which, consistent with its mandate, provided translation services throughout our seminar, ensuring that our Transatlantic dialogue could live up to its full potential; and that the best experts, rather than the best linguists, could be seated at the table.

Just as a reception at the Canadian embassy in the United States had been the highlight of our 2007 seminar, in 2008 an evening at the Residence of the French Ambassador in Washington, D.C., among gilded rooms, venerable paintings and bucolic gardens provided a welcome respite from unconventional and catastrophic crises of all stripes. This event was made possible through our superb working relationship with Dr. Jacques Drucker from the French Embassy. Our thanks go to our hosts, Ambassador Pierre Vimont and Deputy Chief of Mission François Rivasseau; Christelle Piris and her team at the Residence; and to Stephen Flynn, our keynote speaker, whose work is an inexhaustible source of inspiration for all who strive to think intelligently and outside the box about emerging homeland security challenges. We also are grateful for the support of the European Union Commission's Delegation in the United States, and specifically to its Environment Counselor, Malachy Hargadon, who contributed useful information to our dialogue. The Center for Transatlantic Relations is part of the Johns Hopkins University-led National Center for the Study of Preparedness and Catastrophic Event Response (PACER), designated by the U.S. Department of Homeland Security as a National Center of Excellence on Homeland Security. We are grateful for the support of the Department for our work in this area, particularly related to network-based approaches.

There is often an air of artificiality in rounds of applause at the end of a conference, as the question lingers whether the conference itself is being applauded, or the fact that it has ended. Yet during our 2008 seminar one such round of congratulations was clearly as heartfelt as it was well-deserved, when it came to acknowledging the role that our

CTR colleagues Gretchen Losee and Katrien Maes had played in putting it together, and their patience and grace in doing so.

In the end, they, with the rest of our team as CTR, could do no more than provide an overarching sense of purpose and a space for dialogue, with the hope that it would prove as constructive and unconventional as our first discussions had been in 2007. That it did reflects on the quality of our participants, old and new. In addition to demonstrating unmatched expertise, our session leaders helped steer us clear of traditional panel-and-audience formats, to ensure that all could share in the conversation; therefore, as we extend our thanks to Rick Bissell, William Dab, Rune Froseth, Mike Granatt, Patrick Lagadec, Anne Richard, and Jim Young, we also recognize that the success of our collective effort truly lay with all participants involved, as all deserve our gratitude for their contribution. Any added value in the pages that follow is a tribute to them; while errors are my responsibility alone.

Dr. Erwan Lagadec
Washington, D.C.
August 2009

Introduction

The concept of "unconventional crises," or the proposition that they constitute a recent phenomenon, are by no means self-evident. Both tend to elicit pointed questions from those who have not had direct experience of such events, so have not tested first-hand the analytical, let alone strategic or operational legitimacy and value-added of the concept; though this value-added occasionally has been challenged by some who have in fact confronted complex or catastrophic disruptions.

When this push-back doesn't simply reflect a cultural inability to acknowledge emerging challenges and their daunting implications, it is grounded in an incontrovertible point, which in fact is helpful in order to determine the exact meaning that the word "unconventional" must assume if it is to be a relevant concept.

What is not "unconventional" about recent crises relates to the *general* categories of victims, assets, and interests that they have affected. There is nothing new in tsunamis, hurricanes, earthquakes, famines, financial crises, or terrorism; nothing new in human despair, suffering, and confusion; or in polities breaking asunder. Characterizing current events as "unconventional," if it implies willful ignorance of valid historical precedents, is not only self-serving—to the point of being insulting to our forebears—and intellectually foolish: it also surely condemns us to repeat the history of past tragedies just as we claim to have transcended it.

Even quantitatively, though 6 billion human beings on Earth make for an unprecedented number of potential victims of crisis, and assets and infrastructure at risk are both more numerous and vulnerable than ever before (concentrated as they are in disaster-prone areas such as cities or littorals), it would be an inexcusable feat of historical short-sightedness to claim that 21st-century events systematically have had higher consequences than past disruptions. A look back at e.g. the Black Death, the 1755 Lisbon earthquake, the 1900 Galveston hurricane, or the devastation of 1945 Europe easily puts this illusion to rest.

What, then, is so "unconventional" about, say, 9/11, the 2004 tsunami, or Katrina? The answer lies in one word: *networks*; and its most striking implication: a paradoxical combination of *extreme complexity* and *extreme simplicity* in the disruptions that modern networks enable.

The complexity of networks lies not only in the unprecedented variety of stakeholders who hold a legitimate claim to take part in planning, response or recovery efforts; or in the technological sophistication and bewildering interdependence of infrastructure systems; but more to the point, in the fact that not only the *superstructure* of networks (i.e. combinations of organizations or assets), but also their *"lifeblood"* is involved in causing, spreading, and responding to modern disruptions. Not only the "plumbing," but the "water that flows through it." Not only wireline or wireless facilities, but the intangible, nebulous mass of individual callers who will try to reach loved ones in the wake of a disaster, and will immediately raise the response environment to a new degree of complexity if they are unable to do so because infrastructure has failed (as it commonly does in such circumstances). The unconventional complexity of crises that affect modern networks stems from the fact that leaders today must take account of the individual free will, anxiety, irrationality, but also independent response efforts of *everyone* directly or indirectly affected by a disruption—at a time when modern technology implies that all, in a sense, belong in the latter category.

Yet this unprecedented complexity coexists with equally stunning simplicity—or is *identical* with it, the same object perceived from a different angle: the simplicity of societal collapse.

The lifeblood that flows through our systems does not do so haphazardly; millions or billions of individual free wills do not strike their own, aberrant courses; though it appears dauntingly variegated, the maelstrom hides consistent and predictable undercurrents, global dynamics that can emerge, change course, snap in an instant. The main collective dynamics of this kind is *trust* between "leaders" and those they would lead. Trust, however, is notoriously flimsy—never more so than among 21st century democracies. Today's major crises, then, are "unconventional" because responders face the very real possibility that their status as leaders, therefore their entire operating paradigm or "game plan," will lose all validity and legibility *in an instant*; that existing response systems will simply cease to operate; and will lose all traction on the course of events.

The French debacle in 1940 provides an eerie and telling comparison. It was so stunning because it was brought about by the unprecedented, paradoxical combination of two historical currents: the apex of technical complexity involved in military logistics, after several thousand years of continued refinement, coexisted with a strategic state-of-play where instant, utter collapse had been made more likely than ever before by emerging uses of speed and space, such as *Blitzkrieg*. Where French (and many German) commanders had geared up for a new attrition war, they were stunned by the sudden, unthinkable alliance between the apparent complexity of strategic systems, and the simplicity of their sudden collapse. Thus Erwin Rommel, to his surprise, found himself driving his Panzer division unopposed through open fields. Thus crises like Katrina *instantly* overwhelmed defenses in place, as the legitimacy of leaders collapsed with the levees; and wreaked havoc unimpeded among the ruins of failed systems.

"Unconventional" crises indeed, then: because the same old story of famines, plagues, and sundry "horsemen of the apocalypse" now impacts victims and their systems through unprecedented processes. As a participant summarized the point,

> "It isn't that the types of events themselves are unanticipated: but they acquire unconventional characteristics either by virtue of their *scale*; their *frequency*; when you have *multiple causes* at play; and when you see *rippling effects*, and *spillovers*."

Even once the existence of this type of events is acknowledged, a temptation often remains to argue one's way back to a state of denial, by relying on the false comfort of a simplistic equation according to which "high-consequence" events can only be *exceedingly rare*; thus setting a misleading zero-sum dilemma between spending one's time preparing for "realistic, low impact" events, or for nebulous, remote, and "unthinkable" catastrophic crises—as if the latter were the stuff of dreamers, naïve souls in need of a reality check, and trouble-making Cassandras.

The argument is fallacious, for three reasons.

First, by positing a mutually exclusive *alternative* between preparing for either end of the "crisis spectrum," it conjures a misleading straw man: the notion that, somehow, those who underline the risk posed by high-consequence events would have leaders ignore their responsibility to confront mundane disruptions. In fact, it should be made abundantly clear that the opposite is true. Speaking of the "age of unconventional crises" does not suggest that these have become *the rule*, in the sense that all events today are somehow unconventional — a bizarre oxymoron. In other words, it is self-evident that the vast majority of disruptions will remain run-of-the-mill, low consequence events. This, in fact, holds a critical corollary for the arguments laid out in the pages that follow. At all stages the reader should keep in mind that our analyses only concern *unconventional* events: and that the soundness of "traditional" planning and response methods is only questioned here *as it relates* to this specific category of crises. Their validity for more mundane situations is not in doubt; a blanket denunciation of their effectiveness would be unwarranted, and ultimately dangerous.

Second, what we question is the notion that the line runs perfectly straight from the upper left ("low consequence, high probability") to lower right ("high consequence, low probability") corners of the graph that would posit a strictly inverse-proportional relation between the impact of crises and their likelihood. In fact, the *rule* that makes our age that of "unconventional crises" is that they *will happen* with considerable, indeed increasing frequency. At the time of writing, 2009 has added an economic recession and the A(H1N1) pandemic to the already daunting list of e.g. the "mad cow" disease, 9/11, the anthrax attacks, the SARS outbreak, 2003 heat wave in Europe, 2004 tsunami, Hurricane Katrina, and 2007 forest fires in Greece. At some point, a series must be acknowledged as such, rather than as a laundry list of ultimately aberrant acts of God.

Lastly — and perhaps most importantly — even the typical conclusion drawn from the premise that "high-consequence events have a low probability" must be questioned: namely the apparently self-evident, but misleading proposition that, somehow, preparing for such "unthinkable" disruptions is a waste of leaders' time and societies' efforts — including because, "by definition", doing so is supposedly "impossible." First, the "unthinkable" label is often affixed too generously to such crises, indeed sometimes with clear political afterthought, in a desperate attempt to explain away leaders' lack of preparation—infamous examples being the notions that "nobody could have anticipated" 9/11 or Hurricane Katrina, when the opposite is true.

But more to the point: *what if* some events truly are, as of now, "unthinkable"? How does it follow that our leadership and organizations cannot possibly be asked to prepare, or be held accountable for this type of disruptions? The only valid conclusion is that, faced with such risks, it behooves us *more than ever* to address them with enough intellectual audacity to reduce the field of what is "unthinkable"—or rather "unthought of."

Indeed, lest we should fall prey to "zero-sum game" arguments, it should be made clear that spending our energies, *in part*, on confronting the unthinkable will yield strategic insights, operational tools, and behavioral habits that will be relevant, and in fact priceless, when tackling more mundane occurrences.

Yet even if that was not the case; even if collectively opening our eyes to the unconventional, to that which can cause our polities to collapse, was "in vain": still our efforts would have been the exact opposite of a waste of time or resources—as they will have reflected our ultimate *responsibility*: to ensure that our societies will survive, and affirm our solidarity and dedication to that end. In other words, preparing for "high consequence" events is not, or rather should not be an afterthought for leaders: it is at the core of their legitimacy; that from which all the rest follows.

Recognizing that leaders and societies need to tackle unconventional events is a start—a frustratingly elusive start, often—but only a start. What, then, are we collectively to do in order to meet the challenge?

In 2006, the Center for Transatlantic Relations at Johns Hopkins University's School of Advanced International Studies launched the project "Unconventional Crises, Unconventional Responses" precisely to address this question.

Our initial seminar in 2007 began by highlighting strategic and cultural obstacles that must be overcome as a prerequisite for sound analysis and effective action in the face of unconventional events. This ground was covered extensively in the 2008 report by the same title: *Unconventional Crises, Unconventional Responses: Reforming Leadership in the Age of Catastrophic Crises and Hypercomplexity* (Washington, D.C.: Center for Transatlantic Relations, 2007); we will do no more here than summarize its contents.

At issue, then, are:

- the *culture of organizations* (most notably resulting in bureaucratic "silos") — but also the *culture of leaders*, as too many have repeatedly shown themselves reluctant to anticipate the unconventional before it arises, and incapable of thinking out of the box to respond effectively once it does;

- the *identity of leaders*, as a lethal imbalance still exists between the public sector's traditional dominance, and the "subservient" role of private industry, NGOs and the greater public, which fails to recognize their critical input in planning, response, and recovery; while unconventional crises also produce leaders from unanticipated sources and strata irrespective of organization charts.

- *"hypercomplex" maps of actors*, which combine spontaneous coalitions and bewildering mosaics of stakeholders, to include the emerging role of *individuals* as critical drivers or spoilers of response efforts;

- the blurring of comfortable distinctions between "impacted ground zeros" and "*unscathed outsides*," as leaders and responders themselves must realize that they might well be among the first victims of unconventional events. Similarly, these disruptions blur frontiers and prevent linear transitions between planning, response, and recovery, as all three now must be integrated at once into analysis and decision-making.

- the limitations of *planning efforts* that aim to anticipate all potential hazards, and specify for each the behavior expected from every actor: when in fact systemic disruptions will wreak havoc on overly neat and abstract plans in an instant, leaving those whose identity, status, and sense of purpose relied on such guidelines disarmed and rudderless.

In 2008, SAIS invited a broadened field of practitioners and experts from government, private sector, and NGOs, representing the U.S., Canada, France, and the U.K., to move beyond the mere recognition of these challenges, and elaborate practical answers to meet them — indeed, to *test* such answers, or lay out the results of such tests whenever they had already taken place.

The schedule of our seminar, and therefore the contents of the present report, directly reflect this process of maturation.

- In the first place, we threw down the gauntlet of our need collectively to *open our eyes to the unconventional*, based on the example that the loss of critical infrastructure has not been an aberrant side-effect, but a recurring, constitutive impact of major crises, which often fatally undermined preexisting plans that had failed to recognize the point ahead of time. In other words, we explored ways to turn the loss of critical resources and infrastructure into a founding paradigm of our plans, rather than an "unthinkable" obstacle, in order to ensure that workable systems can be rebuilt in spite of such disruptions.

- Second, we highlighted the value-added, across sectors and countries, of a *new analytical framework* that can serve as a basic guideline to recover one's bearings in unconventional crises — though it eschews the temptation simply to replace one set of discredited certainties with another. Based on participants' extensive experience in managing such events, this framework sets out not to provide "guiding answers," but four "guiding *questions*", namely

  A. *What is the essence of the crisis?* Behind comforting labels, chosen either by virtue of groupthink, or because we happen to have a plan for a familiar scenario that we choose to believe the crisis matches, *what are we really looking at?* To what weak point or blind spot in our defensive structures does the crisis genuinely direct its "ramming" or "liquefaction" effect? What interests, though not the most visible, are in fact most at risk?

B. *What are the critical pitfalls?* As noted above, unconventional environments combine considerable complexity with a stunning, instantaneous "simplicity of collapse": so they breed a clear distinction between missteps that will bear no serious consequences, and in fact are unavoidable, and "game-ending" mistakes that can trigger disastrous domino-effects. Flagging these traps is therefore critical: and such red flags should be the first landmarks, the first bearings inked on the new "map" of the unconventional event that responders will draft—most often starting from an otherwise blank page.

C. *Who are the unconventional stakeholders?* Leaders who remain within the comfort zone of their trusted and familiar partnerships will often find not only that they have missed, or stifled, useful potential inputs—but that they have in fact lost all real leadership in doing so, as protagonists with genuine traction on the course of events have emerged elsewhere, among their blind spots.

D. *What game-changing initiatives can be taken* to launch "virtuous circles" in otherwise chaotic environments? The silver lining in the "simplicity of collapse" that characterizes unconventional events is that it is matched by its symmetrical opposite, the "simplicity of salvation": meaning that perceptive and adaptive leaders can stem and even reverse processes of collapse through well though-out and well-timed decisions. All who have lived through and successfully emerged from unconventional crises can point to these rare, but astonishing "miracles at Dunkirk," when responders prevailed against all odds.

- Third, we examined the results of *unconventional crisis cells* which have *embedded in complex organizations* an architecture that lends itself to the dissemination and application, on the cultural, strategic, and operational planes, of the four-pronged framework just outlined. The most successful and conclusive instances have been the "Rapid Reflection Force" set up at Electricité de France; and crisis cell formats at the Civil Contingencies Secretariat in the U.K.'s Cabinet Office.

- Based on an examination of planning and preparedness for flu pandemics—a topic which has been given added relevance and urgency since the outbreak of A(H1N1)—a further session discussed the *practical implications of redrawing allocations of roles and responsibilities* among government, private industry and NGOs—in other words, options for a "new Social Compact": an overarching, consensual architecture which would ensure that initiatives from all three sectors do not impede one another or undermine democratic accountability of response efforts.

- We also proposed a new approach to *resiliency*: first, setting apart "Maginot-line"-type *resistance* (i.e. defense mechanisms located in sections of systemic outer edges that seemingly are most at risk, though the choice might prove erroneous and unhelpfully static) from genuine *resilience*, which implies a system-wide capacity of all components in the architecture to react intelligently and adaptively to unconventional stresses. Second, consistent with the premise outlined above that catastrophic events will fuse response and recovery efforts into a single process, we underlined that resiliency should be built into systems as far "upstream" as possible when laying down the blueprint of organizations (beyond their "crisis management" segments) and their response plans.

- Turning to "complex maps of actors," we then examined the limitations of traditional concepts of *coordination*, to suggest strategic alternatives, and tactical or operational areas for improvement.

  At the strategic level, we explored the notion of *alignment* among international responders: meaning that instead of forcefully and artificially striving to coordinate their efforts—which always elicits push-back when it comes to determining who will be the coordinator, and who the "coordinatees"—intelligent response to unconventional events should rather lay out well thought-out, consensual objectives and norms, *de facto* creating a "behavioral magnetic field": i.e. ensuring that each stakeholder, though working independently or within organic coalitions, will define its remit based on this overarching purpose in such a way that will limit competition and duplication of efforts.

On a tactical and operational plane, the challenge, as Katrina made abundantly clear, often has been to create intelligent systems of "cross-awareness" internationally, so as to break down information – and bureaucratic silos among countries, prevent duplicative or inopportune offers of help, and make sure that traditional *exporters* of aid can also become *importers* should the need arise.

- Lastly, as noted above, there is no doubt that a common prerequisite to achieving these and other goals must be a change in the dominant culture of leaders, prodding them to recognize that preparing for the "unthinkable" is a foundational determinant and implication of the trust invested in them, rather than an inconvenient and secondary adjuvant to it. The next generations of decision-makers must be trained and selected accordingly. Our participants therefore laid out overarching goals and specific pedagogical contents which they suggest elite schools internationally should adopt to prepare future leaders to confront unconventional threats.

The Certainty of the Unthinkable

"Don't ruin the exercise." A participant recalled a training session based on the scenario that the city of Nice, in Southern France, would be hit by an earthquake and a subsequent tsunami.

Nice is, or should be, a perfect exhibit to make the case that the unthinkable is a certainty—and that the alleged "unthinkable" character of some risks often derives from a reluctance to see what is coming, rather than from their unlikelihood or sheer aberration. Tucked in between the Mediterranean Sea and the foothills of the Alps, it is entirely dependent on single sets of critical infrastructure systems: an East-West highway that follows the coastline; and an airport built on reclaimed land at the edge of the water.

To their credit, national and local authorities (after much foot-dragging) have awoken to the risks posed by seismic events in the area; however, the value of their preparation must be questioned when, as our participant pointed out, the premise of the exercise mentioned here was that the airport and highway would escape unscathed from the earthquake and tsunami—though they in fact would be the first assets to be put out of commission; that the Prefect (the high representative of the state in the area) would rely on a crisis cell in perfect working order, all members present and accounted for; and that telecommunication systems would be in pristine shape.

When our participant pointed out the unrealistic, indeed self-defeating nature of these assumptions, the response from organizers was as illuminating as it was problematic: "Don't ruin the exercise."

What this reveals about the ulterior motives, and underlying culture of this training session was made even clearer by a further comment that our participant made in passing during our seminar as he recalled his experience: i.e. not only that rosy assumptions "were" made by the drafters of the scenario, but that, somehow, they "had to be."

This "had to be" says much about what we could call the "cultural sociology" of too many exercises in which the unthinkable is shoved into the dark recesses of everyone's imagination, so that participants can focus on "normal" courses of events with enough peace of mind.

A cognitive analysis would suggest that leaders and crisis managers do not in fact believe that the "unthinkable" can happen; yet this explanation does not hold: as the reaction, "don't ruin the exercise," implies that unconventional contingencies are not ignored altogether, but rather are something of a *taboo*.

It is tempting, therefore, to turn to psychological interpretations: i.e. to conclude that many leaders are simply terrified at the prospect of unconventional disruptions, because they know *all too well* the catastrophic impact that these events can have on the systems entrusted to them. Many who have spent careers trying to convince decision-makers to open their eyes to unconventional contingencies have come to believe that this is indeed the root of the problem. However, while there is some truth to this interpretation—as timorous and narrow-minded leaders have indeed filled the sorriest chapters of disasters and collapse throughout history—it does perhaps not do justice to under-lying, structural factors, and gives too much weight to individual fail-ings—which, if anything, is an intellectual dead-end, as what is to be done once one has called leaders cowards or fools?

What, then, of the structural level? It suggests that reluctance to envisage unconventional threats in plans and exercises stems from the fact that these documents and drills are not, in truth, primarily aimed to ensure the effectiveness of system-wide response in case the worst happens in the future: but to reaffirm in the "here and now" the valid-ity of hierarchies, by underlining *in abstracto* that *leaders would pull through unscathed, and remain legitimate, even if a crisis should occur.* Most exercises, in other words, are not truly geared to prepare an organiza-tion to the chaos of crisis: but aim to underpin the existing order by demonstrating to all levels of the organization that such events *would not in fact be "critical,"* i.e. would not undermine its architecture. That there would be "nothing to see."

This structural reluctance then, projected onto the plane of indi-vidual psychology, at the individual level of leaders' instincts and reactions, can (in some instances) show through under the guise of inexcusable ignorance, or even lack of nerve, *vis-à-vis* unconventional threats. But that is not the sole root of the problem. At issue is the fact that standard exercises and plans *cannot* take account of unconventional disruptions, as those *would* in fact unavoidably disrupt normal mechanisms of leadership and legitimacy, and thus prevent drills and plans from fulfilling their cultural, collective role of symbolically validating the *status quo*. In the case of the aforementioned Nice exercise, collectively opening one's eyes to the likelihood of the loss of critical infrastructure, or to the fact that crisis cell members would be among the victims, would force participating stakeholders to accept that they, and beyond them the central state, would in fact have limited traction on response efforts: *that* is what is intolerable or taboo to the convened officials and experts taking part in the drill, whose own professional status, legitimacy and sense of purpose flowed in some respect from the font of the state's itself. *That* is why insisting on these risks was seen to "ruin the exercise."

And yet, acknowledging the unconventional has become critical today, for two reasons.

The first ties into what we called, in our 2008 report, the limitations of "behavioral plans": in other words, plans that set out to describe a full spectrum of scenarios, and specify for each the reaction expected of all stakeholders at all levels of one or several organizations; thus setting up an ideal chain of behaviors where actions taken by one link in the chain, one level in the hierarchy, flows from, and depends on, the fulfillment by the preceding link of their own crisis objectives. This works well in the face of "normal" events when it ensures a cohesive, organized, and centralized response. Yet it is lethal when confronting unconventional events; as those will wreak havoc on the environment of any number of responders in the "chain," and make their objectives unattainable — thereby immediately precluding other, "dependent" stakeholders from following their own planned course of action. As one or several levels find themselves "check-mate," behavioral plans do nothing but spread loss of bearings, paralysis, and failure across the rest of the organization as through a devastating domino effect.

These domino effects are triggered from the blind spots of "behavioral plans"; in other words, from those scenarios that were not identified beforehand — from the "unthinkable." Therefore, recognizing that it *will* in fact occur would prod organizations to develop and adopt smarter, more nimble, and adaptive "resource-based" plans where unconventional disruptions will be seen as a *foundational premise*, not as an *unrealistic and intolerable contingency*.

This is true especially when anticipating the loss of critical infrastructure; which also hints at the second reason why planning must take account of the unconventional: i.e., most simply, because *it has now become pervasive*.

Collective refusal, for structural reasons outlined above, to envision unconventional disruptions in plans and drills still was—somewhat—excusable at a time when such occurrences were rare. But we have now entered the "age of the (so-called) unthinkable," the age of 9/11, the 2004 tsunami, and Katrina; meaning that a tolerable blind spot—if it ever was—has now turned into a lethal weakness. As a participant noted, human industrial and commercial activities have multiplied risk factors to such an extent that the underlying mathematics in the probability of unconventional events has shifted. This is true, for instance, of epidemiological risks: among an aging and increasingly urban world population, connected by an ever denser web of air transportation routes, regular occurrence of flu pandemics is now a certainty.

So is the loss of infrastructure in crisis environments. Failure of telecommunication networks, in particular, has become a standard feature of unconventional disruptions.

Eight years after the event, 9/11 remains, of course, the archetype of unconventional impacts on foundational infrastructure systems. A participant from the telecommunication company Verizon described how the attacks on New York City and Northern Virginia "represented, really, the 'unimaginable' in this country": highlighting that the company's plans were made instantly irrelevant, other than serving as "a doorstop" that at least opened up enough of a space (precisely because of their irrelevance) to enable committed employees to pull through and save critical systems through sheer courage, grit, and sometimes, bare luck in the midst of tragedy.

Verizon's switching center in Lower Manhattan was located literally across the street from Ground Zero on 9/11. Following the attacks,

Number Seven World Trade Center collapsed onto the Verizon building, rupturing a water main, flooding lower levels, and cutting emergency power. Rubble buried everything up to the fifth floor. Almost 300,000 voicelines went down, as did 4.5 million datalines, including those of the New York Stock Exchange.

Meanwhile, at the Pentagon, Verizon also happened to operate an important switch center. Though fire marshals ordered all employees to evacuate the premises, some set up enough of a coordination mechanism with firefighters and Federal responders to stay on and prevent critical damage to Verizon's systems as water was being pumped in to stem the inferno.

None of this featured in any of the company's existing plans. That it pulled through was a tribute to the capacity of its employees to think on their feet and act with dedication and clarity of purpose, often reflecting their experience of catastrophic events of a different type, namely—in most instances—hurricanes.

The conclusion drawn by a Verizon employee from the experience of 9/11 was that "the way you respond to what was once unthinkable is shaped by how you prepare to what you *can* anticipate." That is true, of course; but converting knowledge, habits, and systems geared for conventional events into a useful arsenal against more unusual contingencies is a difficult process, especially when operating under considerable stress; a process, therefore, which should not be left simply to the skill and instinct of employees, but built into plans and leadership structures.

A workshop among our participants set out precisely to develop practical mechanisms through which organizations, at the structural, strategic, and operational levels, can improve their capacity to anticipate the loss of critical infrastructure, and sustain the effectiveness of their response in spite of it.

First and foremost, organizations should accept, and *make it clear* that the unimaginable *will* happen. On that basis, they should format "routine" drills so that the processes and resiliency that these exercises cultivate can acquire "dual use," i.e. remain relevant in the face of the unconventional; this can only occur through increased tolerance for "out of the box" scenarios that truly "push the envelope." In other words, from a cultural standpoint, organizations should strive to confront the problem with eyes wide open so that the field of what truly is "unimaginable" can be incrementally shrunk through system-wide *efforts of imagination.*

A fundamental adjuvant in this process is the creation of unconventional crisis cells (described in more details below) that will *transcend* the loss of critical infrastructure, and the resulting "stun effect," by being operationally independent from such infrastructure, and culturally "unmoved" by its collapse.

Indeed, it is essential to realize that, though the collapse of *some* critical infrastructure is certain in catastrophic events, not *all* such assets will be equally impacted; so that intelligent, cross-silo awareness, through some form of "virtual registry" of infrastructure in existence and of its ownership, can go a long way towards turning around the problem. This "registry" should also list existing risks, to create a common assessment and consensual prioritization of potential unconventional disruptions and their implications.

This capacity to produce transversal information would also be invaluable in the wake of a crisis, as a *cross-sector assessment team* could take stock of unscathed assets system-wide. Such efforts will require seamless cross-silo communication, therefore considerable efforts towards establishing a "common glossary."

These suggestions make it clear, then, that acknowledging the certainty of the unthinkable, and acting upon this realization, cannot result from top-down dynamics: but from architectural and cultural changes that will involve all strata of an organization, and indeed its environment as well.

This ties back into our earlier remarks regarding the structural roots of leaders' reluctance to recognize and prepare for the "unthinkable." Upper-tier decision-makers will not, cannot of their own volition open their eyes to unconventional threats as long as doing so would imply a fatal weakening of their symbolic status and power, which we suggested is the case at present. The solution to this quandary will not come from the top, but from the bottom. Only when all members of polities and organizations collectively accept that the unimaginable is certain; that they must all partake in preparing for it; that their leaders are not equipped with all the right answers, nor should be judged (or seen to be more or less legitimate) based on their capacity to uphold this illusion—only then will (might?) decision-makers, and especially elected officials, become more confident that confronting unconventional contingencies poses no suicidal threat to their status.

Asking the Right Questions

Acknowledging the likelihood of the unconventional, and the need to prepare for it, only sets the stage for a concerted effort to reinvent, not so much new certainties or knowledge, than a new *strategic posture*.

Unconventional events do not wage attrition wars or siege warfare, but *wars of movement*. What they require from leaders and their advisers, therefore, is the ability to meet speed with speed, think on their feet, be adaptive, and *ask the right questions*, instead of engaging in a futile attempt to dig successive trench lines of supposed "right answers" that systematically will be overtaken by events.

Though some of our participants, when proposing to apply this approach to training drills or actual response efforts, have repeatedly been met with the stale remark that "experts should be answering questions, not raising them," their sustained efforts have resulted in the flagging of critical questions; equally important given the confusing maelstrom of potential unconventional scenarios, those have been "boiled down" to just four which are universally applicable. Though not strictly speaking "bearings" *themselves*, they are initial *leads* that can help recover one's sense of orientation when facing unconventional events, and the ability to map the chaotic environments that such disruptions leave in their wake.

These four questions were outlined in our 2008 report, and again fleshed out in the introduction above.

- *What is the essence of the crisis?*

- *What are the critical pitfalls?*

- *Who are the unconventional stakeholders?*

- *What game-changing initiatives can be taken to recover traction on events?*

Our initial seminar in 2007 had laid out the arguments in favor of selecting this set of questions, and had underlined their value-added in the specific context of Electricité de France's unconventional crisis cell, where they originated. Our following workshop, in 2008, set out to explore the universal applicability of this analytical framework, as we asked our participants to reflect on their experience of unconventional crises through this specific prism.

Strikingly, this single, yet flexible set of analytical principles brought to light common strategic challenges and potential synergies in response efforts *across sectors and countries*, which more conventional approaches would have left in the dark. The following paragraphs will attempt to convey this often stunning sense that the "unthinkable" was being dissected before our eyes, and reduced to its constitutive parts, indeed its "skeleton"; and consequently, that potential mechanisms for cross-silo response were similarly emerging, such as would have remained equally "unthinkable" without our analytical framework.

At this juncture, however, a caveat is required. Even a set of *questions* such as are laid out here can fall prey to the illusion that it provides reassuring *knowledge*, a clear cognitive and behavioral path, as the chaos of unconventional crises makes all stakeholders crave guidelines with such desperation that they are tempted to seize on any "thin red line" to recover the semblance of a comfort zone. The point bears repeating, then, that our proposed analytical framework does not purport to be yet another set of "best practices," or a rigid "how-to" guide. This list of questions results from some of our participants' best efforts to *prod intellectual curiosity, innovation, and flexibility* among planners and responders; it would be ironic if it contributed to stifling them.

Many of our participants, indeed (occasionally drawn by the temptation to play a little mischief on the proceedings of our seminar) took the point and decided to steer clear of our proposed "four questions," electing to use their own interpretative framework instead—as the reader is welcome to do now. Since our goal was to stimulate an open-minded quest for intelligent responses to the "movement warfare" waged by unconventional events, such declarations of intellectual independence also fulfill our purpose.

What is the essence of the crisis?

The danger of premature labels

In the face of unconventional events, labels are lethal.

They will "precipitate" around them, as if around an illusory ker-nel of truth, a comfort zone made up of ponderous hierarchies, pre-ordained plans, and static lines of defense—while the crisis will keep mutating and will thrive on the vast blind zones implied in the label artificially affixed to it. Labels will soothe responders with the false security that they have an exhaustive map of the environment, and trusted guidelines to operate in it; they will stifle curiosity, imagina-tion, and dissent.

The problem is compounded as unconventional crises generally teem with potential labels that seem apparently sensible; indeed that is the whole point: they are so multifarious that any number of "single-word descriptions" will seem to match at least one of their facets—but none will cover them all.

Meanwhile, structural drivers abound that prod responders to pick one, indeed *any one* of these potential labels and "run with it": the false comfort of mistaken "self-evidence"; the assumption that organizations will exhibit a clearer sense of collective purpose if they "know what is going on"; or that a leader's credibility and symbolic status derive in part from his or her capacity *instantly* to "diagnose the problem"; the temptation to pick a label for which a plan already exists and can sim-ply be pulled off a shelf (a bizarre, but frequent reversal in the logic of response); groupthink, when a characterization of the crisis is selected *by no one in particular*, but somehow becomes a tacit consensus among all involved; last but not least, media-driven imperatives, when jour-nalists ask for the issue to be "boiled down" (or is it "dumbed down"?) so it can be conveyed in 24/7 news formats—based on the problematic assumption that the public "will not tolerate complexity."

Labeling crises down

In our 2008 report, we mentioned the risk involved in insidious events: those which, "at the opposite end of the spectrum from iconic crises of catastrophic proportions, are equally unconventional because they remain under radar screens and alarm thresholds, and are prone to be underestimated."

In this respect, the most dangerous label that can be affixed to a crisis—also the most tempting—is one that dismisses it to the dustbin of "conventional," "minor" events and willfully *forces it off* the radar screen—when a different analytical framework would underline, on the contrary, its unconventional disruptive potential, and the urgent need for equally unconventional responses; in the same way that we can overlook the most conspicuous objects in our environment when they happen to be overly familiar and seemingly static.

Among countless potential examples, a participant highlighted collective failures to take stock of rampant low-level violence in some parts of the Caribbean and Latin America, though it slowly eats away the societal fabric of these areas, and therefore holds the seeds of "unthinkable" collapses which finally will set off alarm bells and arouse responders from their torpor—though will do so too late. In the same vein, a colleague mentioned the disastrous state of public schools in some areas of the United States—a challenge which has not always attracted sufficient attention from authorities in the past, or been met with genuinely *unconventional* responses.

The illusion of self-evident characterizations

The surrealist Belgian painter René Magritte is famous for a picture of a pipe to which he added the caption: "this is not a pipe." Unconventional crises similarly tend to belie apparently self-evident and "commonsense" labels, so much so that such categorizations in fact can be self-defeating paradigms of response efforts. The simile with Magritte's art is far from perfect, however: as *moving away from self-evidence* in the case of "unthinkable" crises is not an act of surrealistic provocation, but the ultimate testament to *realism*—such realism as makes it possible to start chasing the prey instead of its shadow.

Katrina provides a perfect example of the temptation to follow "self-evident" labels to one's doom; it also illustrates why the risk is so great in doing so.

It seemed clear enough, as the storm was gathering, that Katrina belonged to that most familiar category among natural disasters: hurricanes—a category 5 hurricane, but a hurricane nonetheless. And yet this assumption, later this operating principle, became part of the problem.

As it turned out, the important point lay in the "category-5" qualification: meaning that a *category-5 hurricane truly isn't a simple "hurricane."* In other words, something more *"emerges"* at that level of intensity, which qualitatively transcends, moves beyond, the familiar set of risks posed by smaller storms. Equally damning for self-evident labels, Katrina was not even a "natural disaster"; it certainly was one in Mississippi: but it was a man-made crisis in New Orleans—again underlining the endlessly variegated, shifting nature of unconventional disruptions. As a participant acknowledged, "Our company had been through the 2004 storm season very successfully—a series of storms in quick succession. We got through that in terrific shape. We underestimated Katrina: we obviously didn't have a real sense of what we were getting into. So it *was* something very different."

Lest Katrina be dismissed as an aberrant case, a participant recalled the "unthinkable" impact caused on the Dominican Republic by the quick succession of Hurricanes David (a category 5) and the smaller Frederic in 1979: highlighting that responders, due to poor access to information, misdiagnosed the most severe consequences of the storms—namely, the spread of infectious diseases due to the breakdown of water supplies and health infrastructure. Thus a "hurricane" had shifted unexpectedly into a severe public health crisis, instantly condemning existing defenses and response efforts to irrelevance.

Nineteen years later, the challenge posed by Hurricane Mitch in Nicaragua proved to hold equally unthinkable ramifications. As torrential rains modified the layout of minefields, local rural communities yet again found themselves surrounded by unmarked unexploded ordinance. A hurricane had shifted into the grim encore of a civil war.

The same *emergence* of hypercomplex and unconventional challenges from among seemingly familiar categories of events past a certain level of intensity holds true beyond hurricanes and other meteorological events. As a participant put it, "we don't know what 'category 5' events are *in general*," where 'category 5' metaphorically stands for this line in the sand that marks a qualitative break in the nature and impact of crisis.

Thus, SARS "wasn't just a 'public health' emergency. Because very quickly you had to develop policies for opening and closing schools; for potentially blocking areas of the city of Toronto; for stopping public gatherings; for running jails; for doing all kinds of things." In other words, the SARS outbreak in Toronto soon came to pose questions for Canadian society that far transcended public health issues, as Ontario for instance "came to deal with issues of racism directed against the Chinese community," which was most affected by the disease. What had begun as a "communicable disease" threatened to morph into a deleterious social dynamic that could undermine the complex edifice of communities' coexistence and integration in multi-cultural Toronto. This transition in the nature of unconventional threats will recur, and indeed has recurred in comparable instances — as post-9/11 suspicions of the American Muslim community unfortunately demonstrate. Similarly, when facing H5N1 from 2004, and again H1N1 in 2009, too many public health or veterinary organizations adopted a myopic characterization of the situation, focusing on its scientific implications when the disruption at hand was societal and economic in nature.

The bombings in London on July 7, 2005 were not in fact a "terrorist attack" in the familiar sense that they would have had a direct impact only on a few assets of physical infrastructure — buses and trains — while causing indirect ripple effects limited to the spread of abstract fear among otherwise unscathed outsiders. As a participant noted, these attacks in fact *directly affected "four million victims,"* as the subsequent collapse of telecommunication systems prevented Londoners from reaching and reassuring their loved ones. From "what if I had been there" or "could it be me next time," the "terrorizing uncertainty" became "was he/she there, and why can't I find out": a much more concrete, personal, and traumatizing proposition. In other words, the attacks were not a localized disruption of the superstructure of networks, but a *sepsis* which spread throughout the bloodstream that flows within them, namely communication: "the instant propagation of dismay and despair."

Food protests that affected a number of developing countries in 2008 involved challenges which "went way beyond the purely humanitarian dimension. We need to look into agricultural production, into keeping global food trade open, and growing use of crops and land for biofuels. So it goes into economic and social issues, into security, and *political* issues."

In the same way, the current economic crisis is certainly not just a "financial crisis"—though an attempt was made, early on, to label it as such with the implication that the "real economy" would be safe from the generally incomprehensible vagaries of Lehman Brothers and its ilk. Nor is it even truly an economic "recession," a characterization which would imply, indeed has implied, overly technical and restrictive responses. It now has trickled down, and out, to involve not only all types of economic interests—but more global and foundational issues, such as democratic trust in all leaders alike: in their competence, sincerity, and motives.

Again, the ongoing war in Afghanistan is not a "war"; indeed the label remains inadequate even if qualified with a myriad DoD mantras such as "irregular warfare," "counter-insurgency," "civil-military effort," or "war 2.0." It is a shifting, often illegible set of challenges that call for a variety of sometimes mutually exclusive answers. As a participant underlined, "stabilization initiatives and capacity-building are almost, in some cases, oxymoronic; resources that you put towards stabilization do not assist with long-term development; and very often, the things that are required for long-term development are antithetical to short-term stability."

So variegated is the Afghan challenge that it uniquely weaves together all four analytical strands in the typology of critical disruptions that we laid out in our 2008 report: i.e. *catastrophic, insidious, cascading, and hypercomplex.*

> "Afghanistan was, in some cases, *catastrophic*: we were dealing with issues of immediate famine in some parts of the country—and yet resources, rather than going completely to support the famine, were also being distributed across multi-ethnic and multi-sectarian lines to prevent exacerbation of violence.

It was *insidious* in some ways: the lack of literacy, and the lack of a civil service existing in Afghanistan was something that—it took us several years actually to realize—was going to hamper and delay our ability to build capacity.

And in many cases, the problems were *cascading*: a response taken today has secondary and tertiary unintended and unanticipated consequences that follow on.

And it was certainly *hypercomplex*: one of the things that we didn't appreciate enough was the ever-shifting role of stakeholders. Because today's donor may be tomorrow's spoiler; and the person who is with you on issue A may be vociferously *opposed* to you on issue B or C."

Self-evident labels most often work against responders not because they entirely mischaracterize a crisis: but even more dangerously—as the fallacy of the description is less conspicuous—because they highlight only one of its consequences, while ignoring others whose impact might be far more devastating.

In 2007, a participant had discussed at some length an illuminating example, namely the "foot-and-mouth" disease that affected the U.K. in 2001; he merely summarized his conclusions a year later:

"The crisis lasted for months, we killed millions of animals, we killed some farmers through suicide, we killed the tourist industry: we killed all sorts of things. That taught us that poor assessment could lead us to protect half of 1 percent of our GDP (the farming industry), at the expense of an industry ten times its size in every respect (inward tourism)."

A colleague described his experience as an aid representative in Dushambe, Tadjikistan, in the mid-1990s, when he had been tasked with tackling border insecurity and Tadjik refugee flows from neighboring Afghanistan. In fact, *in addition* to this dimension of the crisis, he simultaneously had to take account of unrelated humanitarian emergencies, natural disasters, drug smuggling, and pervasive political violence. As in Afghanistan a decade later, these challenges held a nonlinear, indeed sometimes contradictory set of implications for responders, whose bureaucracies unsurprisingly were not set up to bridge those gaps, in part because they had organized their effort based on an over-hasty and simplistic description of the nature of the problem.

An equally illuminating case study was the heat wave that affected western Europe in the summer of 2003:

> "Our biggest mistake was that we misdiagnosed the problem at hand. The first incontrovertible signs that something was amiss came out of hospitals, as emergency rooms were overwhelmed with incoming victims: so that leaders' attention, as well as public debate, immediately focused on ERs' lack of surge capacity. But the real problem was happening elsewhere, in elderly people's homes; and the real driver was their isolation, as they were not properly looked after by their families and neighbors. Eighty percent of all deaths during the heat wave happened at home, not in hospitals."

Even when the characterization of an event switches more quickly from *a priori* to *a posteriori* self-evidence, the initial, over-hasty rush to conclusion weighs heavily on responders as they suddenly are asked to modify their strategic approach and confront an environment that they are not necessarily prepared to handle. Thus, a participant recalled the confusing and daunting impact of a radical change in the categorization of the Oklahoma City bombing in 1995:

> "When we went into the incident, it was a 'building explosion': as we started to respond to it, it quickly became obvious that it was a terrorist attack—one of the first terrorist attacks of significance that we dealt with as a society in the United States; and also in terms of instant media, instant coverage by 24/7 news channels. We had to deal with going from a humanitarian effort to working in a crime scene."

Similarly, a former member of the U.S. Department of State's Policy Planning Staff noted that on 9/11, the meaning of the crisis for her and her colleagues, once the Pentagon joined the Twin Towers among the targets, switched instantly from a challenge to produce prompt analysis of the attacks, to an evacuation situation where their own safety was at stake.

Based on his extensive experience of politically sensitive post-mortem diagnoses, a colleague quickly understood the real "nature of the crisis" when asked to examine how a dozen Columbian lawmakers kidnapped by FARC had met their death, whether executed by the rebels, or caught in the cross-fire of a police assault on their jungle camp. What was at stake in the determination of the truth concerned not only the victims, but the course of ongoing negotiations relating to 50 other hostages held by FARC, including the high-profile case of the Franco-Columbian politician Ingrid Betancourt. A "simple autopsy" could reignite a civil war, and trigger an international incident with France, in light of President Sarkozy's involvement in Betancourt's liberation.

Against technical categorizations: the human dimension

At this juncture, a trend clearly emerges regarding the common, "original sin" of over-hasty labels imposed on hypercomplex disruptions: namely the fact that the categorization of the problem at hand almost exclusively proceeds from purely technical considerations—when in fact it is the *human dimension* that is most challenging, most unconventional, most characteristic of this type of events.

Nothing *per se* prevents the emergence of categorizations of crises based on "human impacts": is a crisis about *uncertainty, loss of trust, despair, despondency, defiance*? But at present the genealogy, identity, and implications of crises, for cultural and organizational reasons, almost always proceed from overly abstract rationales—most notably *law*, and an *asset-based interpretation* of "business continuity."

A participant reflected on the anthrax crisis in 2001 based on this proposition.

> "This was an unconventional crisis, for sure—because of its *psychological and emotional* impact for our staff. The reason was that the situation was *unknown*. With 9/11, we knew what we were facing; the same was true of the 2003 blackout. With anthrax, we didn't know. And our staff were not focused on their work, or anything other than the unknown

threat; so that we, as responders, had to deal first and fore-most with the psychological impact of the crisis."

Colleagues involved in the response to SARS, and in the recall of a brand of soda in France in the 1990s due to (unfounded) fears that the product was contaminated, described in strikingly similar terms the nature of the challenge that these incidents posed, beyond scientific technicalities: namely the deleterious effects of the *unknown*, and the resulting *uncertainty* and *fear*. On this evidence, communicable diseases and biological threats, more than six centuries after the Black Death, and a hundred years after Pasteur, still seem so intangible and mysteri-ous that they elicit intense apprehension, and put collective psycholog-ical dynamics at the forefront of the challenge — even as leaders, when confronting these events, are tempted to address them from the exact opposite side, i.e. armed with the tools of abstruse and remote science.

Faced with the 2004 Tsunami, a major hotel chain instantly took stock of the fact that the crisis was first and foremost a *human* prob-lem — rather than one having to do with physical assets, legal liability, etc. With sparse information and little cooperation from overwhelmed local authorities, the first decision that was made was to repatriate more than twelve hundred patrons who had stayed in South-East Asian resorts of the company's, as well as 250 European staff, in addition to assisting its 500 local employees.

On the other hand, in the wake of Katrina, the same company was surprised to find that the nature of the crisis had shifted towards human emotions and conflict — the emergence, in a chaotic environment, of seemingly "irrational" behaviors such as had never been anticipated by corporate plans. Indeed, evacuees from New Orleans who had been granted emergency accommodation in motels across the region sim-ply refused to leave. The problem was so far off the company's field of vision, which focused on a technical characterization of the chal-lenge, that it only became aware of the issue when a journalist called its leadership with the news that incoming patrons were confronted by evacuees who had overstayed their welcome and yet would not budge.

Categorizing oneself

Labels are more helpful when affixed not to the crisis, *but to one's organization itself.* Unfortunately, precipitous judgments on the nature of crisis are often matched by an equally problematic inability to diagnose with eyes wide open the state of readiness and the relevance of one's own efforts in responding to it. Determining the "nature of the crisis" is no more important than making a sound assessment of "what we can do about it in the current environment." Or rather: the nature of the crisis for an organization can be the very fact that *it is not ready*, or not helpful — that it is part of the problem rather than of the solution.

Indeed, in the final analysis, even the "unconventional" label that we affix to certain crises is only valid because *we* partake in causing them, as we have built up systems with *unconventionally weak foundations.*

> "The main danger in our reflection is to fall under the illusion that what we face is unconventional *per se.* What is unconventional is our inability to take into account vulnerabilities which we ourselves created.
>
> What is unconventional about Katrina is that we had built on flood zones when this never should have been authorized. Take the 2004 tsunami: there is nothing unconventional about a tsunami! They, like earthquakes, have occurred since the dawn of time. What is unconventional is that world population keeps migrating to coastal areas; so that the poles of our global economy are now located in disaster-prone regions. With respect to the current financial crisis, what is unconventional is that banks would ever lend thirty-two times the amount of their reserves. Regarding public health, we should not be surprised by pandemics when more than fifty percent of world population today lives in urban areas. Again, what is unconventional is our inability to wake up to the implications of these trends.
>
> *We are like sorcerers' apprentices, overwhelmed by complexity that we created ourselves.*"

What are the critical pitfalls?

Groupthink and conventional paradigms

Eschewing the temptation to affix premature labels to complex events demands a capacity to take a step back, listen to dissent, open the field of acceptable hypotheses, go back to the facts, and establish the genealogy of emerging diagnoses. In all respects, groupthink is a lethal trap; especially when it occurs among co-opted groups of leaders who, as indicated above, all operate from the assumption that their status depends on their demonstrating superior insight into "what is going on," and would be fatally imperiled should they ever "pause for thought," or indeed for any other reason. As a participant put it, "I spent twenty years as a member of national decision-making groups who sought great breadth of vision by sitting in windowless rooms deep underground, sharing their misconceptions. My greatest asset was therefore constantly suggesting that 'coming out for air' might move things along." Indeed, the same colleague added that "one important component of leadership groups, in my experience, is the 'court jester,' the person who dares to ask 'why,' the maverick who says 'I don't actually believe this is true.'"

Groupthink coalesces around, and builds upon foundational paradigms that result from the accumulated experience of conventional events, which the "unthinkable" often invalidates. So in 1940 French strategy was based on the mistaken premise that the "Ardennes forest was impassable"; during the Vietnam War, the faulty assumption was that "communism formed a single, Moscow-led bloc," blinding the U.S. to the nationalist, independent streak that permeated the V.C. In the same way, a participant noted that in 1918, the Spanish Flu counterintuitively wreaked havoc among the young and the healthy, as would again be the case today with some unconventional flu viruses: the unthinkable, and the ultimate pitfall for planning and response efforts, lay in the fact that "our bodies' defense mechanisms had become our main enemies."

Closing ranks to one's death around mistaken paradigms, in an autistic refusal to entertain alternative interpretations, does not amount to genuine leadership. Nor, however, does an indecisive approach that confuses openness with irresolution. The essence of leadership in unconventional events lies in cultural readiness to subject one's interpretative framework to the permanent test of external input: *but* do so based on a very clear definition of what that foundational framework is in the first place. Failing which, leadership runs the risk of losing control over the *narrative* of crisis, and see its *focus* and *rhythm* hijacked by other stakeholders towards gratuitous debate and blame games. As a participant explained,

> "In the initial stages of a crisis, government typically will get cooperation from the public and the press. People are worried, and they are reasonably compliant, for the first short period of time. But then the critics come out: and the blogs start. So the urge to blame starts very early: and it's very difficult, but very necessary to focus your responders on the notion that: 'we'll get to the criticism later, we'll look back at the events later, but we've got to go through the crisis first: and if we spend all our energy worrying about what we didn't do, we're never going to solve the problem, and we're going to make it a whole lot worse.' But it's very difficult to do."

By losing focus, leaders risk to let the whim of outside narratives dictate decision-making processes. A participant recalled how a health minister had resolved to end a program of vaccination against all evidence in the name of ill-advised reliance on the "precautionary principle," spurred by a recent TV program that had clamored for this decision based on lachrymose interviews with "victims" of the vaccine's alleged side-effects. Failing to develop their own interpretative framework, leaders had decided to rely on a ready-made outside narrative instead, in the process manufacturing a real crisis out of the ghost of one.

To avoid being blindsided by sudden shifts in public narratives that can invalidate leaders' own interpretation, and therefore restrict their legitimacy and margin of maneuver, decision-makers would be well advised to pay more attention to the underlying mechanisms at play in the emergence, ecology and lifecycle of such narratives. As a participant put it, "Today, we suffer from an analytical deficit that only social sciences can resolve, regarding *public perception of risks*: as this should be a crucial element on leaders' radar screen. We must do more work in this field to improve the environment and the effectiveness of decision-making."

Public narratives do not have to be irrational spoilers of response efforts, and can in fact become essential adjuvants, provided leaders pay attention to their underlying dynamics, and undertake concerted efforts to feed facts into the "rumor mill." Thus a participant recalled that

> "People in Toronto initially were concerned when SARS hit; although interestingly enough, once they were educated, they ended up being much more relaxed about the disease than people outside of the city. We found that the level of concern among the public grew as you traveled further away from Toronto."

The difficulty for leaders, then, lies in finding a middle ground between complete "bunkerization" of response efforts, and engagement with outside fields of vision that will not result in a suicidal slide back into the maelstrom of endless public debate over options and performance. The underlying culture that will help leaders find this middle ground can be nurtured, and its development should be a primary objective of training drills—though it rarely is. At the same time, however, it must remain a matter of instinct, and reflect leaders' intangible skills in striking the appropriate balance.

Lethal unintended consequences

The "test" of outside input and interpretations is especially valuable when it highlights that conventional paradigms born of groupthink dynamics hold subjacent but lethal unintended consequences. In 2007, for instance, a participant had made a scathing indictment of WHO's 2003 travel advisory as Toronto was affected by SARS; he summarized his criticism one year on in the following terms:

> "It wasn't scientifically proven, it had never been done before, and it did absolutely no good. What it *did* do was create an enormous amount of extra work for responders, at a time when they had a lot of other things to do; it frightened the

public, and made things seem worse than they really were. And economically, it cost Canada over a billion dollars."

At the time of our 2008 seminar, riots were breaking out in a number of countries due to food shortages; prompting participants to make similar comments against strategic short-sightedness:

> "The worst example of unintended consequences is this 'great' idea that we would make ethanol out of corn; now we've got a shortage of corn, wheat, and rice; and world food prices are going up."

Faced with complex, shifting, system-wide unconventional crises, then, the conclusion is unmistakable: "We've got to think through unintended consequences to a depth that we haven't before; not just grab the simplest straw and say: 'that will do it.'"

Self-defeating plans

The danger in conventional paradigms is also evident on a broader scale: in other words, defensive strategies outlined by conventional plans can become conduits for unimaginable collapse. Unconventional crises thrive in the fault lines, the blind spots of our systems; yet faced with such events, plans can embed blind spots in the midst of our defensive lines: indeed *plans themselves* can become our ultimate blind spot, and be "taken over" by the crisis (just as an IT virus takes over a computer), which then utilizes the "infected" plan as a matrix to spread through the rest of the system. As was the case with the Spanish Flu, our defense mechanisms become our own worst enemy.

This holds critical implications for the mantra according to which "it is better to have a plan, however imperfect, than no plan at all." Certainly this is true in the face of conventional disruptions, when the main—often the only—danger is to cede to anarchy and lose one's defensive shape. Yet when confronting unusual contingencies, responders must be awake to the very real possibility that *their plan might be lethal*—the surest pathway to instant, systemic collapse.

So by 9/11 prevailing wisdom had embedded in plans the proposition that evacuating the Twin Towers held more dangers than staying put. Yet when the attacks occurred, those plans turned out to be the crisis' best ally—conventional planning *fed the problem* as surely as jet fuel did the inferno.

During the SARS outbreak, as in other public health contingencies, plans called for heat monitors to be set up at international airports, in an attempt to identify sick passengers and prevent them from traveling abroad.

> "It doesn't work. During SARS, we screened a million people worldwide; the only case of SARS detected this way was somebody who already knew they had SARS and was traveling to Hong Kong to get treatment. Everybody else passed through airports before they were symptomatic. Once the disease is present worldwide, it isn't going to matter whether it is being spread within the country, or one more patient comes in from abroad. At the *beginning* you want to restrict travel, until it gets into a country, so you can buy a little bit more time. But once it's there and it's around the world, it's just a complete waste of effort. And when it becomes clear that it hasn't worked, the public will be asking why leaders decided to do it. So you undermine public confidence, you use up valuable human and material resources, and you'll interrupt the supply chain, all for something that has no real use."

Equally faulty were plans which dictated that schools should be closed.

> "Sounds easy: but if we close the schools, that means that a part of the workforce has to stay home and look after the kids. And there isn't very good evidence that the decision achieves its goals. It might work in primary schools: but it doesn't work with high schools, as kids simply go to one another's house, or to the mall. Students' education also is compromised, they don't graduate: you get into all kinds of unintended consequences."

Following the 2004 tsunami, an NGO's plan became part of the problem rather than of the solution, as it had failed to anticipate that all thirteen of its country-specific affiliates simultaneously would join the response effort. Similarly, a participant recalled that in the years leading up to hurricane Katrina,

> "Train companies hadn't really thought through what the specific ramifications of their disaster planning were, who the various stakeholders were. One very specific example: we had a plan for evacuating 15,000 people from New Orleans: but every train had to run like clockwork. What's the chance of that happening during a hurricane? Suddenly, you can't move a bunch of people that you anticipated moving."

The most pervasive misconception that will turn plans into part of the problem is the proposition that upper-tier leaders will "necessarily" emerge unscathed from all contingencies: thus suggesting that response efforts can proceed from the top unimpeded. As has been noted, however, the assumption has proven dramatically wrong time and again in unconventional events: triggering "domino effects" through all levels of organizations when subordinates chose to "follow the plan" and simply waited for instructions from above. Equally problematic, indeed, is the assumption that professional responders will also be unaffected, unimpeded by crisis: though 9/11, for instance, provides a tragic example that this is not always the case. In SARS, "We had to take account of the concern of healthcare workers. It was the first time in probably fifty years that they felt vulnerable: that they thought they actually were going to catch the disease, and die themselves, or that they would pass it on to their families."

Worse yet than overly optimistic predictions regarding the availability and status of leaders and responders in the wake of crisis, plans can altogether misidentify the locus or strata from which leadership will have to be exerted if it is to hold any leverage on events—failing to appreciate the complexity of legal and legislative frameworks, especially when responsibilities and chains of command have been dissolved into confusing patterns by pre-crisis political gamesmanship or the inherent tendency that drives organizations towards ever-increasing complexity. The problem is especially visible in federal systems, which combine several layers of government; but it is not restricted to them. Though SARS, in Canada, most acutely affected Toronto, city officials soon realized that their plans had left them exposed, as real authority (and power of the purse) over local hospitals lay mostly with the Province of Ontario—but, more to the point, was scattered among multiple strata, including the national government and international stakeholders such as WHO. In another context, the European Union's best efforts to plan for centralized responses to civil emergencies are undermined by member states' reluctance, in actual crises, to relinquish strategic decision-making, financial resources, and operational assets (as well as the prestige that comes with success) to joint agencies in Brussels.

In the end, extensive experience of military planning led a participant to propose a useful, universally applicable framework to test a plan's validity:

> "When somebody tells me they 'have a plan,' I'm not impressed; and I typically ask four questions to see whether that planning is worth the paper it's printed on.
> Number one: have you held a 'murder board' to question all possible embedded assumptions which may be in there?
> Number two: are the resources connected to the plans? Plans aren't worth a thing if they don't have resources attached.
> Third: will your organization be comfortable with plans morphing from 'contingency-' to 'crisis planning' when an event actually shows up on the horizon, instead of remaining a mere hypothetical?
> And finally: is there buy-in among all stakeholders?"

Loss of trust

Plans are not the only item in our defensive arsenals that can become self-defeating when the "unthinkable" occurs: so can conventional understandings of *the public's reaction to crisis*, and of *the nature of leadership*.

The former need not detain us long; as the dangers involved in presuming that the greater public is naturally prone to panic, and should be fed a rosy picture of the challenges at hand—or simply left in the dark—have been well documented. The approach is suicidal because bad news *per se* is a much less likely and powerful trigger of "panic" than is the public's sudden realization that they have been lied to, and have built their own response posture upon a fallacy. In a world that now combines a dizzying array of potential sources of information beyond leaders' control, this catastrophic loss of trust and bearings will come sooner than ever before. Promising the public "nothing but blood, toil, tears and sweat" counter-intuitively will be more effective in mobilizing public energies, restoring a collective sense of purpose, and ensuring sustainable public trust in decision-makers. A participant insisted, for instance, that in the face of a pandemic,

> "Government experts have got to get the word out; if people *know* what to expect, how many people are going to get sick, who really is going to die, and what percentage, *they will deal with it*, if you give them the facts, and you educate them ahead of time. You keep it simple, you keep it honest, and you keep it consistent. You *never* shade the truth."

Leaders know this, of course; yet seldom exhibit the nerve to act accordingly. During the 2003 heat wave,

> "The French government mismanaged communication. The crisis took place in August; the Prime Minister's 'spin doctors' advised him that 'the French were on vacation, and now was not the time to share disturbing news with them.' So that for four days, the government sent out reassuring messages, though they did not yet have credible epidemiological data."

Ultimately, however, this course of action remains so prevalent less because of leaders' poor appreciation of public reactions, than because of their ill-thought understanding of *their own status* — of the meaning and implications of leadership itself.

When faced with unanticipated crises, leaders will be subjected to a twin set of temptations and fears that can contribute to their doom.

The temptation is to see in the crisis an opportunity to reaffirm one's preeminence at the expense of rivals, based on the simplistic assumption that extraordinary times simplify leadership structures to heighten the status of their very top strata: sometimes indeed result-ing in a "one-on-one" dialogue between "the people" and its "head," along the lines of the mythical narrative of General de Gaulle's "appeal to the French nation" on June 18, 1940. Even democratic leaders will find the prospect irresistible of being "free at last" from any outside interference in this paternalistic conversation with their constituency.

Meanwhile, the fear that weighs upon leaders is that their symbolic status will be irremediably compromised should they fail to culti-vate the notion that the "unthinkable" is only such for lesser souls: that it holds no mystery for them, has not caused them to pause and think anew, and does not question their capacity to make instant deci-sions — reflecting the notion that leaders faced with *unconventional* cri-ses should prove themselves to be equally *extraordinary* in their omnip-otence and omniscience.

Both this temptation and this fear, however, are based on faulty assumptions, and will prove a leader's undoing.

The proposition that unconventional crises will reduce the architec-ture of leadership to the bare bones of a conversation between a heroic father figure and its flock is merely the stuff of legend, the result of too many self-glorifying memoirs. Nobody, in truth, heard De Gaulle's "Appeal" on June 18. As we noted in our 2008 report, unconventional crises, far from resulting in the top strata of power holding (or recover-ing) a monopoly on vision and decision-making, will in fact *spread* lead-ership among a variety of unanticipated stakeholders. We underlined, for instance, that "by the time the President and the Vice-President got engaged on 9/11, the crisis was over! The shoot-down order came down at 10:31 a.m. — almost a half hour after the last plane had crashed in Pennsylvania." Not only the pace of crisis, but also its complex-ity, can affect the role of upper-tier leadership: "In an issue that is as complicated as the SARS outbreak, political leaders usually take a step back: because they don't understand the issues, and they defer to the technical specialists."

Indeed, upper-tier leaders faced with unconventional crises will soon come to the realization not only that they hold little traction on events (at least if isolated from other emerging sources of leadership), but that their legitimacy and trustworthiness compare unfavorably to those of other, unusual stakeholders. As a participant lamented, "we have seen a divorce between elites and the rest of society."

> "A feature of today's crises is the lack of confidence and legitimacy that 'normal' actors can command—politicians, private-sector leaders, traditional media, etc.: as their respective motivations are perceived to be ensuring one's reelection, making profit, and increasing audience levels. At bottom, the definition of *expertise* itself has been undermined, as public opinion will write its own narrative based on poorly differentiated 'relevant voices' irrespective of their actual competence on the issue."

Leaders, then, can endure lethal loss of trust not because they have failed to meet a challenge, but because they are focusing on a *different challenge* than public opinion, as prevailing perceptions of the crisis at hand shift, unbeknownst to experts and established leadership. "The speed of modern communication systems—CNN, but also 'internet 2.0'—creates collective intelligence, collective certainties, based on nothing more than *perceptions*." If leaders fall into this trap through a self-serving understanding of their role, they will contribute to creating an environment "in which nobody can identify who legitimate interlocutors are, who can be trusted on the issues; in which no one will know who leaders are in the first place. In which legitimacy and trust, in the end, will have lost all meaning."

This is not to say that upper-tier leadership must slide into irrelevance in unconventional events—far from it. It will only condemn itself to do so if it misinterprets its proper role in the circumstances, but this is not a preordained outcome. When faced with such disruptions, those leaders can, indeed should play a unique role—though one which bears little resemblance to normalcy, and is certainly not "normalcy on steroids." They must be the *facilitators* of others' efforts to respond on the ground; adjuvants, rather than obstacles, for the process of systemic change that will see unanticipated sources of leadership emerge at all levels of an organization's or polity's architecture. They must be trouble-shooters who clear the path for these unconventional decision-makers.

This does not imply, however, that they must remain in the shadows: quite the opposite. Indeed, while the *ad hoc* emergence of leaders on the ground is an inescapable consequence of unconventional events, is it not *per se* an answer to the challenges they raise; as it does not warrant against a slide into anarchy pure and simple. The preeminence of "upper-tier leaders," then, does not disappear: it simply acquires a new meaning. They remain the only possible source of an overarching sense of direction, the symbolic standard-bearers of collective solidarity, fortitude, and hope, those who will articulate the meaning of the crisis, honestly lay out its challenges, and open up the space for each individual to find his or her own calling in the response. Winston Churchill got part of this fundamentally right during World War II—while also being blind to equally important elements of this approach, as he would not desist from micromanaging strategy and tactics.

Here we touch upon the fallacy of the "fear" that we have just described: the notion that leaders' legitimacy in "unthinkable" events hinges upon their capacity to *do something*, in fact *anything*, as long as it feeds into the illusion of their omniscience. The capacity to identify genuinely fundamental challenges in a crisis, and articulate them clearly so that all can act upon this diagnosis and this sense of purpose, is quite the opposite of "God-given" (or "status-specific") omniscience, and incompatible with the mantra of "action for action's sake." First and foremost, it demands that leaders *think afresh in the midst of chaos*.

Certainly, in the early days of a crisis, the fear that doing so might be perceived as a sign of irresolution or paralysis on a leader's part is not entirely delusional. However, to begin with, leaders can find plenty of opportunities to exhibit their stiff upper lip and resolve for all to see through initiatives that will aim to fulfill the first goal outlined above: namely being the *facilitators* of others' efforts, through legislative or logistical means, rather than by rushing to judgment on the nature of the challenge.

Second, the risk involved in daring to think anew in the midst of crisis is much overstated by leaders obsessed with 24/7 media coverage, and who mistakenly believe that such an effort to collect one's thoughts is a *moment* (which they deem "wasted") rather than a *process*. In fact, confronting unusual crises with the right, "unconventional" approach is a state of mind, a philosophy, a behavioral guideline, which remains compatible with uninterrupted action, decision-making, and visibility—so does not compel the leader to angst-inducing paralysis, or a momentary absence from TV screens.

Third, and most importantly, any potential "de-legitimization" induced through the approach to leadership advocated here pales in comparison to the lethal consequences that have ensued, time and again, from leaders' speaking and acting without a sound analysis of the crisis at hand. As noted earlier in this report, unconventional crises will *simplify collapse*, by reducing "social compact" to the bare bones of a *relationship of trust* between leaders and their constituents. This sets up a "thin red line" that can snap in an instant, and will not be recovered once lost.

Unusual crises heighten upper tier leaders' responsibility *not* to demonstrate omniscience or omnipotence, but to provide a guiding principle so others can act in concert. Only they can do so; as only they can instantly and irremediably lose the credibility necessary to do it, by acting precipitously.

Mismanaging imperfect information

At this juncture, a possible confusion needs to be dispelled. There would be no little irony if our argument were understood to mean that leaders "act precipitously" when they have not "taken the time" to *restore their omniscience*, i.e. to collect *all* relevant facts concerning an unconventional crisis. Trying to do so is a futile exercise in chasing a horizon: a desperate attempt to reassert normalcy by pretending that the unconventional can be tamed, and all its constituent parts catalogued, if only one will pause long enough to gather all the information before one dares to act. This is simply not the case; this is not what we argue for; and the illusion that it can be done is in fact a critical pitfall when confronting such events.

A participant recalls finding himself in a crisis room in Europe, where a simulation was taking place based on the scenario that a dirty bomb had exploded in a major city, while another was about to do so in a neighboring community; and seeing a military officer take charge of response efforts by drawing a matrix on a blackboard, with no fewer than 50 lines and 50 columns, each asking a specific question of the situation. Evidently the officer proposed to wait until all 2500 answers had been filled in before any decision would be made, prodding our participant to suggest that time was perhaps too short to even dream of doing so.

What needs to be "tamed" is not the unconventional or the unknown, *but leaders' fear of it*: their fear of acting upon imperfect information. An "ideal" state of play where all fog of war has been dispelled simply cannot be restored. All "unthinkable" occurrences bring about confusing, ever-shifting environments. Among many characteristic examples, a participant underlined the challenge posed by patchy, contradictory intelligence in the wake of Katrina, most notably regarding the issue of public safety, as uncertainty on that front delayed the ability of companies to deploy staff in order to begin restoration efforts.

The point bears repeating: the intelligent, curious, open-minded approach to unconventional crises that we advocate here is not a *moment*, but a culturally-ingrained *process*, which will enable leaders to make decisions in chaotic environments, looking at maps teeming with *terrae incognitae*, by *continuously*, systematically striving to keep their eyes open to the "unthinkable," to cultivate their imagination, while also setting up basic interpretative guidelines.

Leaving ethical questions unresolved

Among these guidelines, providing answers to fundamental ethical quandaries is paramount. Unconventional crises will undermine the philosophical paradigms of our polities, if only because they will *actually* pose difficult ethical questions that had merely been answered *in abstracto*, or ignored altogether. Simply put, no one else but top elected leaders can appropriately and legitimately resolve such questions, and thereby lay the groundwork for subsequent strategic decision-making and operational efforts. Thus a participant underlined that cross-sector relations could be poisoned, and trust in leadership impaired, through "failure to treat the various stakeholders in an emergency *fairly*."

Of course, in democratic polities, leaders will not make such decisions alone, but should strive to reflect consensual ethical norms; yet in the end, they alone can close debates, sign laws, promulgate executive orders. They alone bear the responsibility—the very definition of "upper leadership" in unconventional crises—to muster the courage and clarity of mind that will enable them to do so. By failing to live up to this mandate, or ignoring it entirely, leaders take the risk of jeopardizing the entire response process, as it will then be based on non-existent or unclear premises which no one else can resolve for themselves. A participant made the case as he recalled his experience through SARS:

"Response efforts have to be undertaken against a backdrop of transparency and ethics. Some of the issues, for example, that Ontario faced were the following:

Could government order, should it order health-care professionals to show up at work? Did it have that authority, within the Acts of Ontario, to hire and fire on the basis of people's willingness to come to work when SARS was in the hospital?

How far should civil liberties be respected, with regard to the sharing of medical information? People are concerned, they want to know who is sick, who is dying: how much can you share, how much can you not?

What do you do about scarce resources? What would we do in a pandemic, where we had a limited number of N95 masks? Where does government step in? Does government step in and seize antiviral supplies that private industry might hold?

Issues such as allocating health care. If you're in the middle of a pandemic, and ventilators in hospitals become scarce: do you abide by a 'first come, first served' principle to determine who gets the ventilator? Or is it the person with the greatest chance of living that gets the hospital bed and the ventilator? And if they get the bed, how long do we give them to get better, before we unplug the ventilator and put the next person on?

These are the kinds of ethical issues that need to be discussed *now*, at local, national, and international level."

Ready-made thought processes

Faced with such daunting questions, temptations abound that entice leaders to desist from an autonomous effort to make critical decisions, and to find refuge instead in preformatted "knowledge contents" and behavioral guidelines. Those seem to hold the promise of a quicker process, when time is of the essence; more importantly, they enable leaders to eschew the responsibility of developing their own interpretative framework, and of living with the consequences of its potential imperfections.

As we noted in 2008, science — or the appearance of it — is the ultimate such recourse, at once providing analytical tools that can yield an overarching interpretation of the crisis; setting behavioral guidelines that will clarify "what to do" in the circumstances; and outsourcing political responsibility not only to respected and conveniently faceless scientists, but more generally to the abstract "Idea of Science," which holds a crucial sway over positivist, Western cultures. This "outsourcing" process out of the realm of politics (hence of political responsibility) is especially drastic as the political and scientific fields are entirely distinct, the latter essentially foreign to the overwhelming majority of the greater public, and to political leaders themselves. As a participant summarized the point, "relying on science is tempting because there's a tremendous urge to do something during an emergency; and it's got to be resisted. You've got to figure out how good the science is: and if the science isn't really good, then don't cling to it."

Closely related to science, technology is another such illusion. As we have seen, during SARS the decision was made to set up costly machines that would screen incoming passengers at airports for signs of illness — a futile initiative, and one that distracted precious resources (logistical and human) from more useful purposes.

The artificial reassertion of normalcy: fighting the last war

The surest recourse to restore one's comfort zone after facing an unconventional crisis, as well as the ultimate pitfall that will compound the impact of its recurrence, is to deny that it has prevailed, or indeed can do so: in other words, to "close ranks around normalcy."

When confronting such events, or planning for the future in their wake, organizations and polities ideally would take stock of the irruption of the "unthinkable" to encourage efforts of imagination that could help shrink the field of what has not been *thought of.* However, reality more often takes a different course, as organizations do not in fact undergo such a cultural reformation. Instead of opening their eyes to unconventional crises—a proposition which they find too unsettling—they choose to see them as aberrations; or simply to extend their definition of "normalcy" *ad hoc* to include, and therefore explain away, the *last* occurrence of the "unthinkable"—therefore condemning themselves to fight the last war when the next unconventional event emerges under an entirely unexpected guise. For instance, a participant noted that current efforts from the State Department and Department of Defense to improve their effectiveness on "reconstruction and stabilization" are based almost exclusively on observations drawn from Iraq and Afghanistan, which will not necessarily be valid precedents to meet future challenges. Another participant eloquently made the same point when he noted that train companies' planning efforts in the years after Katrina

> "became *an 'exercise in having a plan'*; and an exercise that was focused on the commitment that 'our mistakes will not happen again in New Orleans.' But one of the things that we realized very early on about this new plan was: what's the likelihood that you're going to have a hurricane like the one you just had, *again* in New Orleans? And now that you've got trains stationed there, ready to go, what good will they do if the hurricane is in Mississippi, or Jacksonville, or wherever the case might be?"

Worse yet, while culturally validated processes of imagination would highlight the need to enhance interagency or cross-sector cooperation, efforts aiming simply to include the last avatar of the "unthinkable" into existing plans are usually conducted independently within each silo in the bureaucracy, as each strives merely to demonstrate that it has learned the lessons from its last failure. Not only, then, are organizations preparing to fight the last war: but they are doing so by steering their own independent course, without forming an overarching battle line.

Such efforts to reassert the reign of normalcy are built upon an illusion, which the next unconventional event will dispel with unforgiving clarity; meanwhile, this "normalization" process will have stifled dissenting and imaginative voices—the one genuine line of defense against unconventional disruptions. In the words of a participant,

> "I remember, during TOPOFF 2—a major cross-border exercise that Canada did with the United States—trying to convince participants that in our scenario, the resurgence of pneumonic plague, even a small number of victims would bring about a major crisis. And they argued that the situation would not attain unconventional proportions until we had hundreds of bodies. And then, before the exercise got under way, we were hit by SARS! And we found that just a *few* victims drove the whole crisis quite nicely..."

Failures of imagination: the illusion of relevance

As we discussed above, stifled imagination will leave a number of weak paradigms unquestioned within an organization. The worst of these assumptions is the illusion of the organization's relevance and potential traction on events. The problem arises when a stakeholder simply assumes that it can be a provider of help after an unconventional crisis hits, even though it suffers from such a cultural or logistical disconnect with those in need that its efforts are likely to be in vain, or indeed to become counter-productive—condemning the deluded organization to join the ranks of metaphorical Danaids, striving to fill bored vessels with water.

Mistaken appreciation of one's relevance most often occurs when an organization attempts to respond to an unconventional crisis based on its own entrenched habits, processes, and resources, rather than on the actual needs of victims—in other words, when a responder chooses a specific course of action *"because this is what it does."* Thus a participant underlined that international appeals processes in crisis response were not "really based on thorough needs assessment," but on each agency's operational template: leading them to "send the wrong people, and the wrong assets, at the wrong time." Certainly Katrina provides a long, inglorious list of examples where organizations and countries, driven by the best of intentions, yet not by a genuine awareness of circumstances on the ground, ended up "pushing" inopportune offers of help onto the U.S. response system. "Much of the help that came to the U.S. from foreign countries after Katrina simply was not necessary, or went unused." The most infamous example has become the following imbroglio, whose details would make for priceless comedy were the circumstances not so tragic:

> "The U.K. government moved quickly to fly in 500,000 humanitarian rations, or Meals Ready to Eat, to help feed people in the American South. And then the U.S. Department of Agriculture ran after these rations and tried to collect them all up, because they were afraid of spreading Mad Cow disease. And so, many of them were collected, especially if they had meat in them; they put them in a warehouse, they didn't know what to do with them, a whole bunch ended up being buried, it was a complete waste of 2 million dollars' worth of food; some of them were sent overseas again, crossing the Atlantic for the second time, to be fed to border guards in Moldova and Georgia."

In this instance, the illusion of relevance was nurtured among foreign donors by mixed messages stemming from various U.S. agencies—reflecting differences among their respective culture and objectives. Indeed, while the State Department proclaimed that no offers of help would be refused, FEMA, on the ground, simply did not believe that any assets from overseas were in fact necessary.

Discussing Hurricane Mitch, which hit Central America in the fall of 1998, a participant recalled that

> "The problem was, in the early phases, we did not have any good needs assessment: we didn't have diagnostic tools—the Office of Foreign Disaster Assistance and USAID were not typically concentrated in that part of the world, they had a lot to do elsewhere. So in the early phases we get into the routine of folks in Washington asking: 'well, what do you really need?' and the folks on the ground saying: 'we don't know, send whatever you can.' And that's a dialogue of the deaf which makes life difficult."

A colleague broadened the argument by arguing that

> "We must make sure that impacted local communities
> remain at the center of their own response plan: that they
> are empowered, and have the skills and the knowledge to be
> able to *control* the supplies coming in, so the help coming in
> these communities is demand-driven, based on their needs
> and their response plan, not supply-driven by forty differ-
> ent organizations trying to provide them with assistance
> that they may or may not need."

The same tendency for each organization to act in accordance with
a narrow definition of its own remit also prevents them from developing an understanding of the "big picture" at stake in an unconventional event. This causes another critical pitfall: namely the risk that
no one responder, or no coalition among them, will attempt to tackle
the full spectrum of disruptions caused by such a crisis, or endeavor to
diagnose the "natural history," the root causes of the problem—thus
condemning every stakeholder's efforts to futility.

Organizations that fail to reinvent their own *unconventional remit*
based on an imaginative assessment of the unusual demands brought
about by unconventional events run the risk that the crisis itself will
force upon them an unanticipated shift in their identity and mission. A
participant described how her hotel chain underwent this exact, traumatic process in the wake of Katrina:

> "Evacuees in our motels had been in the Superdome in
> New Orleans; they had nothing: no food, no clothes, no
> money, and nowhere to go. The bus comes, drops them
> off: eight people to a room, for months. *And so we became a
> social agency.* We had to worry about food for them; we had
> to worry about communications; when was the next time
> that we were all going to hear that they had to be out in
> a week, and they get very upset, they call the media, they
> call me: and it just became this very chaotic, volatile situ-
> ation. Where could they get aid? We were constantly, at
> Corporate, providing them information, in their particular
> market, where they could find housing, permanent hous-

ing, where they could find food, medical help, all of that
sort of thing—and pushing that out into our motels, which
are a very basic business structure: it's not complex, but you
add on top of that becoming a social agency, it became very
complex indeed."

Stovepipes and blind spots in partnerships

A final critical pitfall when facing unconventional events lies in the
risk that organizations and their leaders will be blind to the emergence
of unusual stakeholders—or will include these newcomers in fundamentally unchanged, thus ineffective partnership structures—due to
legal or regulatory pressures to stick to trusted partners and formats,
or simply to the force of habit. This tendency typically results in a state
of play that a participant described as "*ad hoc* coordination mechanisms
that just don't work, because they don't include the players who should
be a the table: or worse, they include players who don't understand
their roles and responsibilities; or even worse than that, who *think* they
have a lead role but don't, and really have nothing of value to bring to
the table."

This, in fact, is the combined consequence of falling into several of
the traps outlined above: namely being overly hasty in "pulling a plan
off the shelves"; and mistakenly believing that unconventional events
will not reshuffle the "architecture of leadership" or the allocation of
roles and responsibilities, when the opposite is true.

The implications of this risk are well-known, and will not detain us
here—in part because they were discussed in more detail in our 2008
report. *Stovepipes*, which in "normal" environments ensure the coherence of response efforts and a common understanding of allocation
of tasks, will now become lethal impediments to information-sharing
across organizations and countries; narrowing their respective understanding of the environment affected by crisis, and therefore leading
to duplicative, predatory, inopportune, even self-defeating initiatives.

At this juncture, the question is rather *how* to avoid this particular
trap, and prevent such blind spots when drawing the blueprint of *ad hoc*
partnerships in the face of unconventional events. This introduces the

third major question outlined above among our proposed interpretative framework.

Who are the unconventional stakeholders?

Of course, the word "unconventional" as applied to planning and response partnerships is relative. Considerable evidence worryingly suggests that, for the public sector, the word still would apply to the notion of balanced, respectful, and fair working relationships with private industry and NGOs. Most participants from national governments acknowledged that, even today, they "still had a *lot* of work to do to bring in the private sector."

Certainly, undeniable progress has been made on this front since, for instance, not a single representative from either of those two sectors was invited to take part in the Hurricane Pam exercise in 2004, an omission whose catastrophic implications were made clear just a year later when Katrina hit the Gulf Coast. However, much remains to be done if inclusive efforts on the part of the public sector are to turn from belabored and unnatural exceptions to the rule, as often seems to be the case at present, to a culturally ingrained and self-evident habit. Simply put, if progress is not made on the fundamental prerequisites of cross-sector cooperation and mutual awareness, the recommendations that follow will remain futile—as, more importantly, will current efforts to plan for and respond to unconventional events.

"Unthinkable" crises will entirely reshuffle three "ecosystems" to the point of making their internal makeup, structure, and dynamics, as well as their systemic interconnections unrecognizable: namely those of response stakeholders (*leaders* and *spoilers*), victims, and "relevant observers."

Two processes, or undercurrents, contribute most notably to this metamorphosis:

- A "surge to quantitative extremes" on the spectrum of potential stakeholders, as relevant actors become at once *everyone*, and *unusually small groups* of individuals—even sometimes individuals themselves. This can bring about the organic emergence of unanticipated coalitions, in ever-shifting patterns that teem with dialogues of the deaf and fleeting overlaps of otherwise unrelated interests.

• Qualitatively, a brutal "differentiation of relevance" which heightens the role of *unanticipated critical constituencies*, when they happen to find themselves at a vital node (or bottleneck) in the response efforts, and thus turn into unlikely leaders, spoilers, or at least kingmakers; while at the same time other stakeholders with a strong *a priori* claim on preeminence find the "rug of leadership" pulled from under their feet as the map of the emerging chaotic environment marginalizes them against all likelihood.

The few and the many

We have already highlighted the risk that responders will mischaracterize an unconventional event by taking into account only one of its variegated consequences. This in turn weighs upon the identification of the most important category of stakeholders in any crisis—yet, strangely, one whose real demands and needs are often misconstrued or ignored: *victims*. Blind spots that obscure certain dimensions of a crisis on responders' radar screens result in an equally selective definition of the identity of its victims, and restrictive appreciation of their numbers.

This is all the more problematic as unconventional events tend to produce system-wide impacts—meaning that disruptive or traumatic dynamics spread and trickle down throughout organizations and societies: therefore, they often involve unusually large numbers of stakeholders, so much so that the challenge for organizations might not lie in the unconventional *identity*, but in the sheer *numbers* of partners and victims.

So on 7/7, as we noted above, not just the passengers injured or killed in the explosions on buses and trains were in fact victims of the terrorist strikes: in a striking "rush to quantitative extremes," the crisis impacted four million Londoners who could not call and reassure their loved ones due to the breakdown of cellphone service.

From a private sector perspective, the same quantitative jump translates into the fact that, following Katrina—or any other unconventional crisis—

> "Stakeholders were our *customers*—where we dealt with new paradigms regarding the notions of 'service' and 'rapid response'; and our *employees*—the first priory was, 'where are they, where are their families?' So 'stakeholders' took on a very different meaning with Katrina."

In 1979, labeling hurricanes Frederic and David as conventional weather events condemned a whole swath of the Dominican Republic's population to the unenviable status of "forgotten victims": those who were hit not by winds or waves, but by the subsequent breakdown in sanitary conditions and water supply.

The challenge for responders, of course, is to avoid falling prey to a facile version of the proposition that "everyone is a victim" in unconventional events, which would prevent needed efforts to prioritize among impacted populations. System-wide disruptions and traumas should be acknowledged; but this does not dispense responders from digging deeper to identify the groups and individuals most at risk; it is merely a prerequisite for doing so intelligently.

This dialectic between the many and the few holds true not only for victims, but also for responders. For a start, just as everyone seems to be a victim in certain unconventional crises, so everyone can become involved in response. Following natural disasters, for instance, "social mobilization can be extraordinarily quick, and entirely outstrip needs assessment and existing processes for the inflow and the staging in of supplies." In the wake of the 2004 tsunami, "NGOs that rely on public donations rather than government funding were unprepared for the size of public interest, the size of public response. This in fact raised critical issues for them in terms of how they could manage expectations, the incredible amount of money that came in, and the resulting risk to their reputation, all of which exceeded what they were used to."

Yet there is more to the problem than the sudden irruption of innumerable stakeholders in response efforts. More crucial is the unconventional relationship between them and minute groups of participants who happen to hold crucial sway on events — not however *by themselves,* but through a symbiotic relationship with *everyone around them.*

Our 2008 report described at some length the insightful observations drawn by a participant from the case-study of the fuel protests that brought the U.K. to paralysis in 2000, most notably with respect to the remarkable influence that small groups, or even individuals, could hold on the unfolding and the resolution of an unconventional crisis. The same colleague only summarized his remarks one year on, as we will do here.

The point is not only that "three hundred protesters brought the British economy to its knees in four working days." The matrix of the crisis was rather a simultaneous rush to opposite extremes on the quantitative spectrum of potential responders (from the individual to the societal): as this *small group* found itself at a critical node in the system, and wielding a disproportionate power upon it, not because of its own status, resources, and initiatives, but because of the way *British society as a whole* reacted to their behavior. "They picketed our refineries — and in one case, they didn't even have to picket the refinery, they just said they were going to": desperate hoarding of gasoline by British consumers did the rest, and indeed precipitated the crisis, in *a destructive symbiosis between the many and the few.*

This combination of quantitative extremes raises a formidable challenge for leaders, who can only recover traction on events and collective behaviors if they find ways convincingly to communicate *at once* with everyone, and with minute groups endowed with entrenched identities, worldviews, and vocabularies. This instantly sets "official" responders, in particular the state, in a position of dependence: as they must rely simultaneously on the news media, and on individual, largely autonomous relays within small relevant groups.

The link between the many and the few as interdependent responders or spoilers in unconventional events is so tight that neither of these two approaches to communication holds priority over the other, and neither will be effective if the other is ignored. Certainly, the same observer of the 2000 fuel protests in Britain concluded that "there is no greater force in the nation than the collective opinions and behavior of citizens; and the state's only effective weapon in this particular circumstance—and many others—was effective mass communication." Yet he also recalled that the resolution of the crisis only came when a single *individual* convincingly relayed the state's—and more importantly the public's—growing impatience among the handful of protesters who picketed refineries.

Thus, "the relevance of everyone" calls upon leaders—most notably, but not exclusively, in government—to weave an intricate web of balanced and mutually beneficial relationships with a great variety of stakeholders. A participant underlined that

> "The Department of Homeland Security has done a good job of recognizing—though it sometimes was *forced* to recognize—that it's not just government leaders that need to be involved; it's the people on the ground, it's the community leaders, churches, companies, business, small businesses…: everyone needs to have a say in how we prepare and how we respond."

A colleague from a non-governmental organization recalled being less successful in dealing with this "explosion of stakeholders" in the wake of the 2004 tsunami:

> "A critical pitfall for us was the number of non-traditional players that were suddenly in the field. In most emergencies, we're used to working with the government, with the UN, and with other major international NGOs: but suddenly we had moms and dads, and small NGOs, and church groups, private sector, and the help of government departments that weren't used to being involved in emergencies: all suddenly in the fray; and there was a huge amount of extra coordination that was required."

This quantitative surge to the extreme in the number of relevant stakeholders brings about structural challenges: for though unusual actors may be involved in response efforts (or strive to be), traditionally dominant responders in government and elsewhere still hold sway over the legal and logistical conditions of their contribution. Following unconventional events, the problem has focused especially on the issue of access to impacted areas, and specifically of *credentialing*. This remains in the hands of public-sector responders, whose generosity in handing out credentials directly reflects their understanding of the identity of valid stakeholders: resulting in the exclusion from response efforts of potentially precious contributors — though some might also be unwelcome impediments or outright spoilers. Adequately drawing the line is a difficult challenge — which is considerably compounded when government fails to realize that the problem exists in the first place.

On a broader scale, the dialectic between the many and the few translates into the familiar proposition that an unconventional event that affects a specific locality or region will hold implications for other countries as well. A colleague noted that the terrorist attacks of July 7, 2005 in Britain also had an impact overseas, as transit systems in large cities everywhere scrambled to advise their safety officials, as well as their customers, on the exact nature of the risk, and the most effective way to respond to it. In the same way, the Afghan turmoil affects "victim states around the world: victims of terrorism, victims of the drugs produced in Afghanistan": while all regional powers, including bitter enemies such as India and Pakistan, hold the keys to a resolution of the crisis.

This presents a specific bureaucratic challenge to government. Domestic agencies such as DHS remain in their comfort zone, culturally, legally, and organizationally, when they set out to create working relationships with a broad spectrum of stakeholders within their own country. Yet, the same participant who commended DHS on this front added that

> "On the international side, we're still hampered, as our system still tends to rely on traditional international structures and leaders, and diplomatic relations. So when we come across situations like gang violence or organized crime overseas: leaders might not be the ones who have information on that, or have the ability to affect it! It may be a local church somewhere that happens to know — or to have some sway on — someone who can do something about it. But again, that's still beyond what the U.S. government have been able to accomplish so far."

Differentiation of relevance

Unconventional events will leave chaotic, unrecognizable environments in their wake in part because they will undermine traditional understandings of stakeholders' respective relevance in response efforts. Unlikely categories of actors will suddenly become paramount, while others, correspondingly, will see their assumed prominence vanish.

Two different, indeed contradictory dynamics contribute to this phenomenon, as the unconventional makes criteria of "relevance" at once simpler, and more complex.

For a start, unconventional crises will confront all victims and responders with life or death situations, reducing their appreciation of priorities to the bare bones of the urge to save oneself and one's family or friends first. A participant explained that on 9/11,

> "The role of families became apparent: for example when my colleague in the next office no longer was 'the analyst on financial crisis issues,' but turned to me and said: 'I'm a single mom, I *have* to get home': *my mission* became getting her home."

Yet, as we have seen, such events will also bring about unusually complex sets of stakeholders, whose relative importance will be equally unconventional, as the crisis makes "normal" leverage mechanisms ineffective and compels the emergence of alternative combinations and hierarchies among responders and observers.

For instance, following the Oklahoma City bombing, non-governmental organizations, which had been used to interacting with donors, volunteers, and victims, suddenly had to come to terms with the dominance of a new category of stakeholders: the law enforcement community. In the wake of Hurricane Mitch in 1998, the road to recovery in Central America unexpectedly ran through U.S. congressional districts with large Hispanic communities, which prodded a bipartisan effort from their representatives in Congress to raise resources and awareness in order to respond to the crisis. The 2004 tsunami often forced local authorities and Western embassies in the region into a state of paralysis; their relevance for the executives of an international hotel chain was fatally undermined, as the company instead turned to new, unanticipated working relationships with European ministries of foreign affairs, tourism, and justice, port and airport authorities, airline companies, even psychologists. In the same way, the circumstances of a participant's enquiry into the death of Columbian lawmakers—which we described above—were so unconventional that Presidents Sarkozy of France and Hugo Chavez of Venezuela became unlikely protagonists in the process.

Typical in this reshuffling of the relative relevance of partners (or potential spoilers) is the sudden and unsettling irruption of the "new media" on the radar screen of organizations unused to this form of nebulous, anarchical scrutiny—or to potential loss of control over the diffusion of their message, and its interpretation. Indeed, the implications of the sudden leverage that web-based sources of information acquire in unconventional crises led a participant to argue that "a study of the mechanisms of public communication among different demographics and across different populations ought to be part of any effort to think anew about crisis management."

Turning from societal to local factors, unconventional crises will suddenly heighten the relevance of charismatic individuals who can muster enough trust to organize impacted communities—from which initial response must stem—so they can metaphorically put their "fingers in the leaks of imperiled dikes": community leaders, family doctors, religious leaders, etc. "So when communications are in jeopardy, government should brief those people, continuously. They should be identified and 'mapped' ahead of time."

This "differentiation of relevance" in part proceeds from a "differentiation of impact," as unconventional events, instead of a ground zero surrounded by an unscathed outside, create a complex combination of "infected" and "resistant tissue": thus leading to the paralysis of trusted partners, while other stakeholders become capable of unanticipated contributions to response efforts.

The determining factors in these variations of the scale of impact among different constituencies often remain puzzling. However, a clear rule of thumb applies in many instances: since these events affect *networks*, differentiation in their severity will depend upon a population's distinctive reliance on specific network systems. Thus, a participant highlighted that following Katrina, text-messages often were the only usable function of cellphones. This instantly created a chasm in the effectiveness and fluidity of communications between adult and younger victims, reflecting cultural differences in their respective familiarity with text messaging.

However, vulnerability in the face of unconventional crises can stem from much more traditional factors of discrimination among certain strata of affected populations, in terms of status and resources. As a participant explained,

> "When you get to the ground, there's not 'one' community of victims, and we need to be very careful not to talk about people as if they all have the same interests and the same needs. People are differentially impacted by disasters: we know that women are often more affected; very poor people and vulnerable people are more affected—Katrina is a classic example of that."

This analysis of unanticipated fluctuations in the respective relevance of stakeholders should not, however, suggest that they can only remain passive when faced with the unconventional, or that their capacity to respond effectively is a matter of pure chance. Reasserting responders' control over their own fate "against the gods" is precisely the purpose of the fourth question in our interpretative framework.

What initiatives can be taken to recover traction on events?

By definition, we cannot provide an exhaustive overview of such initiatives, which are as variegated as the unconventional situations they aim to confront. There would be a clear contradiction in proposing to lay out a list of "good ideas," a new "body of knowledge" that would simply replace a set of static plans with another. The value-added of the following remarks, then, lies rather in highlighting the common, subjacent *thought processes* that led responders to identify unconventional initiatives; and the categories of strategic challenges on which they focused their efforts to launch "counter-attacks against the unconventional." Two such categories emerged during our seminar, cutting across sectors, countries, and specific situations: coalition-building, and the recovery of time.

Creating unconventional coalitions

As we noted above, unconventional crises will thrive in the interstices of defense systems and the blind spots of radar screens: yet they are not so apocalyptic in nature that they do not themselves have soft underbellies, or cannot be flanked. Exploiting these opportunities places unconventional demands on responders, as they must extract themselves from the comfort zone of their trusted alliances and partnerships, which now provide useless, indeed sometimes suicidal defensive trench-lines. Instead, they must reinvent coalitions that will be as unusual as the crisis itself, joining forces with partners who find themselves located at complementary nodes in the system; and together rebuild a complete field of vision so they can attack the weak points in the "system of crisis."

This, of course, is entirely dependent upon a sound assessment of the question that we have just addressed, namely the identity of unconventional stakeholders, and their respective relevance. An open-minded, imaginative evaluation of the protagonists in the field is a critical prerequisite if an effective coalition is to emerge. A participant from private industry acknowledged that

> "Major corporations tend to rely on a certain trusted circle of friends for intelligence and support; it is not that we are *suspicious* of those beyond that circle, but we are concerned about working with them. And we need, as a corporation, to break out of that mold: as it doesn't work when you're dealing with an environment like Katrina."

Thus, when striving to spread epidemiological data out among responders in the wake of Hurricanes David and Frederic in 1979, a participant realized that the most effective conduit to do so would not be the local government, but the national Red Cross.

When the Murrah Federal Building in Oklahoma City became a crime scene in 1995, NGOs ensured that they could work in symbiosis with the law enforcement community by "developing quick response teams that could work in this type of environment, that were pre-cleared: people that had experience in working with the law enforcement community, could speak their language, and could advocate for the organization."

After Hurricane Mitch in 1998, a silver lining in the destruction of Central American crops was that it freed up commercial cargo ships, which found themselves with nothing to export, and were therefore available to transport aid from the U.S. to the affected areas; these ships were all the more valuable as the U.S. Department of Defense's airlift capabilities had been severely dented by a concurrent operation in Iraq. So it is that the State Department and USAID came to strike a partnership with private cargo ships specialized in the banana trade, rather than with their somewhat more conventional partners in the Pentagon.

When confronting the SARS outbreak in 2003, airport authorities in Canada saw the need to create an unconventional coalition among relevant stakeholders, setting up a platform within the airport where they could exchange information and coordinate decision-making. As a participant recalled,

> "We were particularly hampered because the federal agency that was the authority of jurisdiction for quarantine had relocated off the airport a couple of years prior to the situation: so there was absolutely no infrastructure in place for stakeholders to coordinate their mandates at the airport. Therefore, the airport authority became the administrative arm of this effort: we had to think outside the box in order to set up this structure in very short order. There were over 120 experts and/or authorities that were looking for a place to work out of at the airport. So we quickly assembled with their representatives to coordinate some type of communication mechanism; and in the absence of a public health structure, what we ended up using was an established crisis management model which we tweaked a little bit to make it work in this particular situation that required flexibility."

The United Kingdom provides encouraging examples of structures that resemble the cross-silo systems that our participants advocate. In 2003, the U.K. updated its civil emergency legislation with a new act that drew in a variety of stakeholders as emergency responders. The resulting mechanisms now include local and central government, private utilities that deliver critical infrastructure, and emergency services. Some of these fora meet and work at regional and local level. Indeed, when London was hit by suicide bombings on July 7, 2005, the local structure, "London Resilience," played a critical part in ensuring a successful response. Regular preparatory meetings slowly have broken down barriers among silos, including government's traditional reluctance to share decision-making powers and access to information: "Actually, we found that business and NGOs had been very keen to engage with government. And although the British government still suffers from a surfeit of secrecy, these local relationships have supplanted much of the mistrust that had been there."

Response efforts undertaken by New Orleans' airport in the wake of Katrina especially stand out among unconventional coalition-building initiatives that enabled leaders to recover traction on events against all odds. As the airport was turned into a helicopter hub, a shelter, a field hospital, a morgue, and a military base in the wake of the storm, the airport staff instantly had to learn to interact with the military, medical personnel, and victims—and do so with no communication capabilities.

Though faced with different circumstances, a colleague also reached across silos when he struck "an unusual alliance" with the Organization of American States, and came to operate directly under its Secretary-General, in order to steer clear of the sensitive political implications of his medical enquiry into the death of Columbian parliamentarians: helpfully combining "political understanding with our scientific effort on a multi-disciplinary basis."

A participant summarized the point in these terms:

> "We want a governance system that can harness the energies of non-traditional partners, and their skill sets. And even in case there is no partnership established pre-disaster, we want to have a system that can bring them into the response organization, so they can work with us."

This quote, however, illustrates a potential pitfall in the interpretation of "unconventional coalitions." Government especially is so used to dominating cross-sector partnerships that it might understand the point to mean that its existing networks simply must be broadened to include unusual, yet "junior" stakeholders. In the face of unconventional events, this is a recipe for failure, not only because it will artificially stifle any genuine contribution from incoming partners, but also because they will not find the government's offer to support its efforts in a subservient position particularly tempting, and will simply decline it. If government fails to realize that not only the make-up, but the internal balance within cross-sector coalitions must change, it will soon find itself a general without an army.

This paradigmatic change is especially critical if upper-tier stakeholders are to take the final, critical step towards the creation of unconventional coalitions: namely joining forces with *the population* itself. Certainly, a participant from the public sector pointed out that "people are a lot more resilient than we think, and we can harness their energies, and they can do a lot of good." Whether this can happen, however, depends on the meaning one gives to "harness." Simply endeavoring to "*tap into*" individual energies and resources will not work, and plans to do so will only sound good as long as they remain untested. What is needed is genuine empowerment of private citizens' and local groups' initiatives, based on a "two-way street" relationship with government such that representatives of civil society can take part in planning and decision-making, and information can travel both ways in times of crisis.

Following the 2003 heat wave, France developed "the first epidemiological plan that was truly cross-sector, rather than narrowly focused on ERs." This was based on the paradigm that

> "Once people even *reach* the ER, *it is already too late*: they *will* die. Epidemiological data on heat waves unambiguously shows that our priority must be to act before victims need to be transported to a hospital. In other words, we must wage our battle in people's homes. Yet if we are to do so, hospitals and doctors suddenly lose their monopoly on response: we enter others' remit, the Red Cross, networks of volunteers, social services in small towns."

In the wake of the 2004 tsunami, a hotel chain demonstrated the potential value-added in creating such unconventional coalitions between upper-tier leadership and private citizens—or in this case, employees—based on a culture of empowerment that enabled them to operate independently with full, tacit support of the leadership structure, and an approach to information sharing that combined top-down with bottom-up exchanges.

> "The company was able to put together teams of volunteers who for instance would staff call centers. Some of our employees abruptly returned from their vacation to join in the effort. They would also greet repatriated victims at the airport—large teams comprising more than 40 volunteers each, which we put together at the last minute, from nothing. So we created a genuine volunteer structure within the company."

Similarly, Katrina yields valuable examples of unconventional coalitions that came to involve private citizens, and crucially benefited from their input:

> "For all the bad news about Katrina, still remarkable initiatives were taken on the ground; notably involving local communities, NGOs, associations, faith-based groups, educators…: and youth! Young people were among the most innovative: they helped thousands of victims; they came up with solutions that did not feature in any plans, that nobody had ever thought of."

The point is not so much to "play the hand you're dealt," but to identify *what winning "hand" can be put together* from a confusing set of cards that are not specifically "dealt" to anyone. A participant with extensive experience in the war-torn Balkans and other crisis hot spots explained that

> "Typically, our plans were irrelevant to the situation on the ground. And when I was sent over, I would be told: 'beware that you'll be dealing with the worst of the worst, the situation is intractable, and there's no way out: so just do what you can.' But once in theater, I would make do with the people that I found there; and produce 'virtuous circles' that plans

hadn't anticipated, through bottom-up approaches; striving to recover the lineaments of control over the situation, upon which the rest could coalesce through positive emulation."

In the end, a participant summarized the argument most clearly when he argued that

> "This is where we should direct our efforts in the face of unconventional crises: how to produce joint responsibility, how to create linkages, set up shared intelligence, enable cross-fertilization of ideas and initiatives: and how to do so as quickly as possible—as the discriminating characteristic of today's crises is their pace."

In this effort to build up unconventional coalitions, the media are of course critical, as the most powerful cement that can ensure collective mobilization. This suggests that intelligent coordination with, or "alignment" among media outlets is paramount when confronting unconventional situations. Even the oft-decried new media, such as social networking sites, can turn from potential spoilers—which threaten to deprive leaders of all control on relevant voices and prevalent narratives—into a critical asset, for two reasons: first, because their inherent speed can keep up with the pace of unconventional crises; second, and equally importantly, because they cut across "silos of media users," thus enabling responders to reach a broader variety of potential stakeholders whom they would want included in emerging unconventional coalitions.

Regrettably, prevalent culture among the public sector has not always awoken to this potential. Thus, when facing the 2003 heat wave in France,

> "Government made a critical mistake in managing partnerships: very quickly, it came to consider the media as the enemy, because they publicized the views of whistleblowers, and were deemed to be 'pouring oil on the flames.' Yet this was *par excellence* a situation which demanded that government strike an alliance with the press, as doing so was crucial to mobilize the public, rekindle solidarity, prod people to visit seniors and encourage them to take in fluids."

The attitude decried here is but an avatar of the frequent paradigm that the media, whether new or old, necessarily will be *spoilers* of
response efforts—thus laying upon them the "burden of proof" that
they have more noble intentions when societies face unconventional
crises. A participant flagged this flawed assumption as a major structural risk in Western democracies, and called for a cultural change in
perceptions of the media's input: "It is essential that experts strive to
educate the media. They are no more obtuse or self-interested than
other stakeholders. When you convince them that they can increase
their audience by taking a responsible stance, they do it. Opposing
decision-makers to journalists *a priori* is facile and unhelpful." Indeed,
a colleague noted that the United Kingdom (in a cultural context
perhaps more conducive than others to such solutions) has set up a
successful structure—the "Media Emergency Forum"—to engage
a constructive, balanced conversation between government and the
news media with the aim to think through the implications of unconventional events for public information; resulting in a system whereby
government can utilize news channels to put out information, while
making no claim on editorial contents—thus separating "information" and "news."

Skillful reliance on the media, in fact, can help meet another challenge that threatens to impede innovative coalitions: namely the apparent paradox that their unconventional makeup must not reach such a
point as will make them unrecognizable in the eyes of other stakeholders and the greater public. As a participant underlined, "well-estab-
lished brands are very powerful in times of stress, because people turn
to the familiar. During the terrorist attacks on London in July 2005,
the BBC website received 1 billion hits before its stopped counting."

The same dialectic between the unknown and the familiar holds
true beyond public communication. Thus, following the 2004 tsunami or Katrina, the surge of well-meaning individuals who traveled
to the affected areas to contribute to response and reconstruction
efforts, in the process building up unconventional partnerships, could
not have been successful on its own—and indeed could have become
self-destructive—had it not coalesced around the more familiar Red
Cross, Oxfam, or Habitat for Humanity. This suggests that the need
for unconventional coalition-building, far from marginalizing established stakeholders, simply entails that these trusted actors themselves

must contribute to such partnerships—though without necessarily *initiating* them.

Recovering control over the pace of crisis

Unconventional disruptions will often lay claim to the *space* in which responders operate, making it entirely unrecognizable. There is not much that organizations can do about this, other than open their eyes to the fact that they now find themselves "behind enemy lines," in a profoundly alien space, a territory that they no longer rule. Yet responders must and can fight the crisis on another terrain, another dimension: *time*.

The impact of unconventional events will threaten to make responders' time as chaotic as it does their spatial surroundings. As a participant put it,

> "It's very difficult for responders to know where they stand in a crisis, including *vis-à-vis time* itself—because the conjunction of the time of the organization, the time of decision-making, the time of partners, and so on, is very confusing."

Yet even more importantly, crisis will *suck time out* of decision-makers' environment; it will impose its own, frantic pace, "moving a lot faster than traditional response mechanisms can handle"; it will also dictate a chaotic, anarchical, brutal *rhythm*. This indeed is the main, the most daunting breakdown that the unconventional brings about: loss of control over one's own time—over the definition of common timeframes, the management of time pressures, even the allocation of rest and shifts.

The most valuable initiative that decision-makers can take to recover traction over the course of events, then, is one that will push back against the "time of crisis," and reassert, at least in part, stakeholders' control over chronology and pace, setting up what a participant termed "robust, *rhythmic* decision-making systems."

In practice, successfully fighting the crisis for time translates into triaging the issues that it raises both in terms of their *importance*, and of their *scope*: so that responders can produce a recognizable remit and rhythm for their upper-tier decision-makers, asking them to resolve *only* those questions which are especially pressing, and also pertain to a "strategic middle ground" between the overly remote "big picture," and the granularity of obstacles on the ground.

Finding this twin middle ground to triage issues with the right *urgency* and *import* demands that two mechanisms be put in place:

- Genuine empowerment of responders in the field, so that practical obstacles that they confront can be resolved on the spot without being sent up the chain of command, clogging it up, and breaking down the rhythm of upper-level decision-making;

- Meanwhile, a specific crisis cell must be tasked with keeping its eyes on the big picture, on contingencies "beyond the horizon," and feed its assessment at appropriate intervals into upper-tier leadership: thus providing "agreed assessments of facts and options that will force decision-makers to consider the whole picture—not wallow happily in the defense of their separate interests."

This, in fact, is the exact purpose of the unconventional crisis cells that Electricité de France and others have put in place, and to which we now turn our sights.

Unconventional Crisis Cells

Overview of mechanisms and concepts

Electricité de France: Rapid Reflection Force

In our 2008 report, we described at some length the unconventional crisis cell that Electricité de France has set up to train for and confront unusual disruptions. Its name, a spin on the mantra of "Rapid Reaction Forces," hints at its underlying paradigm: namely that when confronting the unconventional, *rapidity* and *reaction* are not enough—indeed can be self-defeating—if not underpinned by a deliberate process of equally unconventional analysis and horizon-scanning. In such circumstances, instead of rushing towards premature or inopportune action, based on mistaken assumptions and inadequate plans, and papering over the cracks of angst-inducing loss of bearings among decision-makers, the g*enuine priority* is to think on one's feet, be imaginative, ask the right questions—and do so under considerable time pressure.

One year on, this tool has been refined; its architectural linkage with the rest of the company's crisis management framework has become more mature (and culturally ingrained); and, more importantly, it has proven its worth in a number of training drills and actual events.

Before we summarize our seminar's conclusions in this respect, however, a caveat is in order. Leaders at Electricité de France who have tested this mechanism do not presume that they have found *the* answer to the management of complex events; or that it is universally applicable to other companies, other sectors, indeed other national environments. They are not "selling a product." They come to the issue not as the guardians and promoters of some organizational Holy Grail, but from a keen awareness of the underlying strategic challenges posed by unconventional events. Exhibiting a self-satisfied, corporatist proselytism, from a company that deals daily with the potential implications of nuclear accidents, would not only be out of place, but foolish.

A participant described the genesis of the "Rapid Reaction Force":

The first signal that alerted EDF to the emergence of a new type of crises was the "millennium storm." While crisis managers' and the public's attention alike had focused on "Y2K," the "millennium bug," France in fact was hit by two hurricanes that crossed the North Atlantic and impacted EDF's entire network in December 1999. Three million clients lost power, and one of the company's 58 nuclear power plants was flooded. This was a situation which EDF never had anticipated. It took them more than a month to restore service to all parts of the country. This was the first, traumatic sign that they could be confronted with contingencies for which existing plans, processes, and organizations were entirely inadequate.

Many of the unconventional crises that have affected part of the world on a yearly basis since this first salvo have specifically impacted EDF's interests, or been too close for comfort. 9/11 highlighted the vulnerability of critical infrastructure; during the terrorist attacks on London on July 7, 2005, a bus was blown up right across from one of EDF's headquarters in the city, injuring some of their staff; the 2003 heat wave, when 14,000 died in France, put in question the operational and safety norms of EDF's nuclear plants; Katrina's impact on local utilities held sobering lessons; urban riots that broke out in the suburbs of several French cities in 2005 were triggered by the death of two youths in one of EDF's substations; while the avian flu, and now H1N1, hold critical implications for the company's management of its workforce.

In the end, EDF has come to the realization that, far from being aberrant, unfortunate, or unrelated occurrences, these incidents demonstrate that the company has become a broad target for emerging disruptions, due to the nature of its profession and its international footprint. This assessment in turn has helped focus minds on the need for the company to rethink its planning and preparation. The implications of such crises are too formidable simply to be ignored, even in purely pragmatic, business terms—as insurance costs, for instance, have skyrocketed from one event to the next.

EDF's characterization of unconventional events shares much with the analysis laid out in this report. They occur in an increasingly complex environment, involving a growing number of stakeholders; instantaneous exchange of information worldwide (whether through the internet, or 24/7 news channel that thrive on conflicts of opinion and contradictory assessments among self-proclaimed experts, in the process blurring everyone's bearings); and the growing role of critical networks, such as telecommunications, electricity, natural gas, petrol, etc. — indeed, electrical power often is the common denominator of network disruptions, as nothing can go on without it.

This emerging picture suggests that crisis management mechanisms of earlier decades, which served us well until the end of the 1990s, today have become increasingly ineffective, and that we must change our approach to crisis response. In this context, Electricité de France has set up a new tool: the "Rapid Reflection Force." Two years on, it has become part and parcel of the company's crisis headquarters, and disseminated a new culture of crisis management.

Organizationally, this mechanism has been added onto an existing setup that combined a logistical crisis cell; another unit in charge of crisis communication — media outreach, drafting of communiqués, etc.; and at the very top of the structure, a cell tasked with strategic decision-making.

Within this framework, the RRF has been a *pool* comprising about thirty members who have exhibited the capacity to confront unconventional, potentially traumatic situations with a stiff upper lip, while also being available at short notice. They combine a variety of profiles, which exist in every large company of this type: including sociologists, communication experts, former directors of local sites, accountants, etc. Among them, five or six will be called upon in a given situation: so that the exact makeup of each team is never the same — yet always strikes a balance among imaginative "thinkers," and pragmatists who can translate their intuitions into workable proposals.

Their collective purpose is to feed into other crisis cells a *different outlook*, one which transcends the pressures of operational crisis management, and eschews traditional processes and approaches whose validity is questionable when facing unconventional events. They ensure that the head of crisis response efforts retains an awareness of the "big picture" — which overwhelming demands on his/her time and leadership would otherwise preclude — based on the paradigm that an organization cannot successfully respond to or recover from unconventional crises if its field of vision does not include a system-wide appreciation of challenges "beyond the horizon."

In other words, the RRF is a spur that will prod crisis leadership to *keep moving*, keep thinking, never indulging in trench warfare against unconventional disruptions—as such events will instantly overwhelm or turn round all attempts to draw static lines of defense or restore intellectual comfort zones. With this objective in mind, the critical weapon in the RRF's arsenal turns out to be insightful questions, rather than preformatted answers, which are the building blocks of artificial certainty, the Trojan horses of instant collapse. As we noted, for instance, the analytical and strategic framework highlighted in the preceding chapter (our "four questions") emerged from the RRF's experience.

In addition to describing the RRF's makeup and remit, it is essential to underline what the RRF *does not do*, in order to dispel misgivings that can greet the emergence of such unconventional structures, due to entrenched corporatist interests, or a mistaken understanding of the object at hand—indeed occasionally disingenuous misunderstandings, as some have indulged in contrived straw-man tactics to push back against the innovation.

The RRF *is not* "one more ponderous bureaucratic layer." It remains a small, nimble structure—and more importantly, it fills a genuine gap, providing a tool upon which the very survival of a company or polity might well come to depend when facing unconventional disruptions.

The RRF *does not* imply the "outsourcing of legal responsibility" away from legitimate decision-makers; its aim is not to take "wicked problems" off the plate of those in charge of tackling them. More to the point in democratic contexts, it *does not* create technocratic "philosopher-kings," as it does not imply that faceless "experts" somehow take over decision-making from elected officials. The purpose of the RRF is to *contribute* valuable information and assessments into the decision-making process, not to *hijack* it.

The goal of the RRF's "critical initiatives" *is not* simply to make corporate or other leadership "look good." The RRF should not be confused with a clique of "spin doctors," or a presidential campaign's "war room" monitoring blogs to nip all and sundry rumors in the bud. When facing unconventional events, such an approach would be self-defeating. The team does not work for the "greater glory" of the upper strata of an organization; it is not a praetorian guard that closes ranks around the emperor when the barbarians are at the gate. It helps the company to recover traction on events, not simply to salvage a brand or a bottom line (though those are not trivial objectives), but because it makes a pragmatic, sobering assessment of the dangers involved in unconventional events, and recognizes the ultimate responsibility that major organizations and their upper-tier leadership hold in effectively meeting those challenges.

By now, the Rapid Reflection Force is much more than an inchoate exercise in institutional tinkering. Since 2005, it has been tested successfully in a half-dozen crisis exercises—based on a broad spectrum of scenarios, from avian flu, to the loss of IT capabilities, breakdowns of the electric grid, or incidents in power plants. It has also proved its value in three "real life" crises.

Certainly not all of these drills and incidents have amounted to unconventional, let alone "unthinkable" events such as have been described throughout the present report. Some might indeed seem relatively mundane. If anything, this suggests two remarks that highlight the RRF's value. First, it is encouraging that its input has been sufficiently acknowledged throughout the organization for crisis responders to utilize the tool even when the stakes are seemingly limited. Second, and more importantly, the successful "downwards spread" of the concept shows that even seemingly routine events can hold unconventional implications, when they occur—as they increasingly do—in complex environments. These incidents can emerge within EDF, but trigger domino effects beyond it; responders will rarely avoid media or political pressures altogether; moreover, as a state-owned company now opening up to private capital and EU-wide competition rules, EDF has had to learn that rival utilities eager to seize upon instances of vulnerability will always cast a shadow upon the management of apparently "internal" incidents.

Indeed, the RRF most spectacularly proved its value-added in a crisis whose unconventional nature lay precisely in the catastrophic consequences that would have been brought about by "under-labeling" the contingency as a "non-event."

In the space of a few months in 2007, a number of EDF employees working at a nuclear plant committed suicide off-site. The deaths could have been dismissed as unfortunate yet unrelated incidents which did not *directly* involve EDF, as they had not occurred on the premises of its plant: while attempts to describe the suicides as a *series* that held implications for the company's work environment could have been ascribed to "troublemakers" yearning for the media spotlight, and exploiting the tragedy in ongoing power-struggles. The temptation also existed, for EDF's upper strata, to consider the situation as a purely local problem which did not belong on its agenda.

The RRF, however, enabled EDF to eschew groupthink, and opened the company's eyes to the global environment—most notably the emergence, among public opinion, of an interpretative framework that could fatally undermine the company's credibility if it persisted in a dismissive state of denial. Indeed, the issue had taken "a life of its own" which transcended the specific case of EDF, as clusters of suicides had also occurred among other major corporations in France: resulting in a heated public debate on work conditions which tapped into public resentment of "arrogant bosses" and "inhumane capitalism." In this context, public attention was especially focused on "flagship companies" that combined high brand recognition with a typically French status as "standard-bearers of the French socio-economic compact"—also "coalmine canaries" warning of underlying societal problems: all of which EDF epitomized. The RRF helped the company understand that it had now come to "stand for something else" in public conversation. Whether it liked it or not, its every move was going to be scrutinized, simplified, caricatured, to reflect dogmatic representations feeding into the broader argument. Simply put, EDF ran the risk of becoming the face of "evil capitalism." The immediate manifestation of this came in the form of local and national media swarming the vicinity of the nuclear plant and EDF headquarters in search of "witnesses" who would corroborate the dominant narrative.

Paramount among "lethal traps" were decisions that would lock the company into a static defensive posture based on denial and arrogance. Culturally, EDF's upper strata might have been most at ease with a purely legal approach to the series of suicides, indulging in an arcane disquisition of its responsibility, or lack thereof. This however was a language that other stakeholders were not ready to hear, and which would have irremediably turned public opinion against EDF. Whether or not the suicides had taken place "off site" was beside the point; the company's leadership could not simply wash its hands of the matter.

Taking account of the broader environment highlighted the critical role of unconventional stakeholders who otherwise would have remained outside EDF's field of vision. Of course, they included the families, but also the tight-knit and distraught communities of the deceased; more unusual was the role of politicians who happened to be running in the French presidential election at the time, and vied to position themselves in the raging debate over work conditions, the nuclear industry, and capitalism's evils by making definitive statements on the nature of the problem and generously apportioning blame, without necessarily exhibiting much concern for the facts.

Critical initiatives that would enable EDF to recover traction on events similarly flowed from this broadened awareness of the environment.

The RRF insisted that corporate leadership give unmistakable signs of its concern for the situation: as noted above, it did not do so for "cosmetic" reasons, but to prevent company-wide, indeed societal breakdowns that would ensue if such initiatives were not forthcoming. In the event, EDF's president sent out a senior delegation on-site, tasking them with meeting all employees (irrespective of their personal or professional relationships with the deceased), trade unions, medical staff, for a substantial period of time; thus enabling leadership to collect precious insights into simmering concerns *vis-à-vis* work conditions and the company's evolution—but more importantly, resuming a healthy conversation through all layers of the company, permeated with shared concern for its welfare, rather than poisoned by internal rivalries, mistrust, or facile recourse to class warfare.

This initiative stopped, indeed reversed ongoing or impending domino-effects: most notably it vented out mounting internal pressure—rather than putting an artificial lid on it—and deflated the media frenzy around the case—again, a positive outcome *not* because leadership simply "fooled the media" into hounding another prey, but because it gave the lie to the conflict-laden narrative that had attracted media attention in the first place.

Cultural and organizational challenges remain to ensure that the RRF takes root within EDF. Though actual incidents or training drills have convinced participating upper-tier leaders and crisis managers of its value-added, the company still needs to develop a "general culture" of unconventional events that will permeate all layers of the organization, and will turn unconventional responses into a matter of collective instinct. Structurally, the linkage between the RRF and other crisis cells must be further clarified, so that all stakeholders may develop a clearer understanding of what can be expected of the mechanism—and what cannot; as well as fine-tuning the *timing* of RRF input into decision-making, which is essential to its effectiveness. In addition, the profiles of RRF members are so uncommon that the underlying "pool" of contributors can only be nurtured and expanded through sustained training efforts. The format of the mechanism itself can yet be improved, as our participants showed when they put forward several suggestions. For instance, a colleague argued that the team "should give more say to members of the general public: we could envisage setting up a group of civil society representatives that the team could consult, in order to test its proposals and insights on the general public"; while another participant advocated a permanent RRF that would remain active in "peace time," though under a different guise—turning into an "analytical cell" that would scan the environment for *weak signals*, the crucial implications of which might otherwise go overlooked.

Lastly, as noted above, EDF is under no illusion that it has found a perfect answer to unconventional challenges, or indeed that *any* mechanism restricted to a single organization can claim to be effective, when these events affect much broader environments. The paramount structural and cultural challenge, then, lies in prodding international, cross-sector dialogue on the issues at stake, with the aim to develop equally intelligent and nimble response mechanisms on a broad scale, cutting across bureaucratic silos and national borders.

Afghanistan: "intellectual swarming"

Lest EDF's experience be dismissed as one specific to the private sector, or France's cultural or regulatory environments, another participant used strikingly similar terms when describing his own efforts to trigger unconventional thinking in a theater that could not be further removed from European electrical grids and nuclear power plants: international reconstruction and stabilization efforts in Afghanistan. He also underlined the bureaucratic and cultural limits of his endeavor in ways that highlighted, *a contrario*, the value of EDF's Rapid Reflection Force.

> "We were hampered by a cultural antipathy to new ideas. What we had, as an analogue to EDF's RRF, was something we called 'intellectual swarming': it was a brain-storming session where everyone was invited, and no idea was a bad one. But there's not an appetite for that kind of work, perhaps, within some established bureaucracies, and so you find that the entrepreneurial good ideas are not well received and are not funded. We had to come up with a 'good idea cut-off date': we had to say, at some point, 'we have to stop thinking through the issue, and we've got to *spend money*. That was both necessary for operational reasons, and to meet the expectations of the Afghans and the world: but it's also a fatal flaw in an unconventional problem! Because when you stop *thinking* about the problem, you create the second, and third, and subsequent *unintended consequences*."

Based on this experience, the same participant described the type of unconventional cell that he argued should exist in every leadership structure:

> "For every action that we put on our whiteboard, I would want to run it by this team, and say: what would an enemy do? But equally important: what are the unanticipated consequences that we didn't think of? And this team would comprise members from every sector of government and society, all of whom can contribute something from out of the box. And they would be looking for the things that no one else thinks of. Because a number of things that I saw

on whiteboards had consequences that were worse than the curative that they were offering."

Mapping networks: "hubmasters" and "hubwatch"

EDF's Rapid Reflection Force has no monopoly on ongoing efforts to develop unconventional crisis cells that can feed critical information into upper-tier leadership and broaden its field of vision in the face of unusual crises. It is merely one incarnation of a set of ideas whose compatibility—indeed overlap—across a variety of organizations in different countries results from the fact that these stakeholders are facing comparable challenges, and strive to learn from one another.

Thus, in a British context, a participant has developed a set of notional structures whose objectives are broadly convergent with the RRF's, though their respective vocabulary might differ.

The proposal stems from the paradigm that organizations faced with complex events will have to navigate chaotic environments built up of unconventional and endlessly shifting *networks*. The mapping of emerging stakeholders, risks, opportunities and constraints, without which leaders' efforts to respond to the unconventional are doomed to fail, therefore must start with an understanding of relevant networks, and of the organization's position among them. Our participant, then, argues that "every organization should have somebody who understands its role within networked society as a hub. We call these people 'hubmasters.'"

These hubmasters cannot succeed in mapping system-wide complexity if they remain isolated in their respective silos. Across sectors and countries, then, they themselves must weave a web among hubmasters: a *network of network-watchers*, a coalition of mapmakers. This would not only ensure that they can acquire relevant information when faced with unconventional disruptions: it would also enable them to "create and facilitate a culture of interoperability" among their respective organizations when the unconventional occurs. "They would be seeds for a change of culture, in which organizations learned the value of cooperation in times of stress."

The case for "horizon-scanning" and "red teams": unconventional training exercise

As noted above, training drills have been as powerful as actual incidents to make the case for unconventional crisis cells—yet only as long as these exercises themselves remained unconventional. This of course is a critical caveat, as the vast majority of training sessions merely aim to test participants' knowledge of a pre-set plan which purportedly "holds all the right answers," thus turning the drill into a ritual confirmation of existing hierarchies and certainties.

More effective are training exercises that aim to raise questions instead of validating answers; and do not shy away from pushing participants out of their comfort zone, while conveying a realistic sense of the set of pressures that will weigh upon responders when the "unthinkable" strikes. A critical mechanism to achieve this is to group participants into several teams, both because they in fact would have to work in partnership with others when facing actual events, and because such a format prevents the exercise from turning into a succession of individual, magisterial interventions where each leader in turn takes the floor to explain why he or she would react with unmatched skill and control in a particular situation—all the while paralyzed by the fear that their peers or subordinates might come to the opposite conclusion.

Participants in our 2008 exercise thus set up four teams:

- "Political leaders"—"in charge" of response efforts due to legal frameworks and cultural expectations, though their effectiveness depends on transcending this cultural perception to understand that other stakeholders are equally relevant.

- "Civil society"—representing NGOs, private industry, public opinion, local communities, and concerned individuals.

- "Rapid Reflection Force"—tasked with bringing a broad appreciation of the environment to bear on leaders' decision-making.

- "Red Team"—thinking "on behalf of the crisis," in other words scanning defense systems and response efforts for interstices and weaknesses in which the crisis could thrive.

The main purpose of our scenario was to combine realistic, indeed *anticipated* or past incidents into a maelstrom whose unconventional nature lay in its very complexity: so that the main challenge for responders would be to map the environment with enough intelligence and flexibility to cut through the "fog of war," prioritize issues, and prepare for movement warfare against unavoidable shifts in the situation's dynamics, as some issues would subside while other acquired critical mass.

In addition, our format compelled participants to organize themselves, discuss their options, and make decisions *with too little time*, and *too little information*, both of which are hallmarks of unconventional crises.

The specific make-up of our scenario is anecdotal. Suffice it to say, it combined vague yet ominous threats from al-Qaeda; a suicide bombing on U.S. soil; the first, confusing signs that contagious diseases, including a new, Tamiflu-resistant strain of flu, might be spreading out of Muslim Asian countries into Western hubs; while bank transactions were affected by disruptions of the SWIFT system, and French and British banks gave signs that they might be nearing collapse along the lines of Argentina's recent financial meltdown. Further crowding responders' radar screen, seismic tremors were detected under Yellowstone's caldera; unusual sunspot activity affected telecommunication and military satellites; and a new conflict arose between Gazprom and Ukraine, threatening interruption of natural gas delivery to Western Europe.

A substantial list of issues, then: yet one which upon reflection undeniably comprises a realistic combination of events—so realistic in fact that some of these incidents at least have actually occurred simultaneously in the recent past.

The essence of the crisis

Because of the complexity and variety of the events at hand—itself an accurate reflection of the real-life "noise" that confronts responders, though many exercises will artificially lay out an environment reduced to a single disruption—the essence of the crisis lay not with any single aspect of the scenario, but with leaders' capacity to *organize their radar screen* and make sense of it. Failing to do so is a death sentence, as the pace of crisis, and an anarchical collection of emerging "relevant voices," will then gain the upper hand over response leaders.

In this regard, the Rapid Reflection Force, or equivalent unconventional crisis cells, provides a unique asset, in the shape of an "extra set of eyes" that creates multi-layered and flexible options for crisis managers in their effort to build up situational awareness. In the face of complex, confusing series of events, "organizing one's radar screen" tends to imply a rigid selection of "relevant" or "pressing events," while incidents not deemed to belong in this category fall by the wayside entirely, thus broadening the organization's "blind spot." The RRF enables crisis managers to create a field of vision that is as complex and multi-faceted as the crisis itself—indeed an "intelligent network of radar screens"—as leaders can task this cell with monitoring certain sets of issues, and feeding its assessment back into the decision-making process when the need arises: thus ensuring that this monitoring is not simply "outsourced."

This however leaves crisis leaders with the difficult task of determining appropriate criteria for the selection of issues that belong in their own, immediate field of vision. Based upon our scenario, participants highlighted three such guidelines, which clearly have universal value. They focused on

- Disruptions that hold international or national implications—while others should be left to local authorities, until they come to "pull" national assets back into their own monitoring or response efforts.

- Events upon which upper-tier crisis leadership can in fact exert influence—meaning for instance that geological phenomena in our scenario were seen to be secondary.

- Events which *"hit the general public closest to home,"* and thus can trigger societal breakdowns and collective loss of cohesion and trust. Communicable disease, disruptions of the banking system, and loss of telecommunications were deemed to be paramount in this category. While crisis leaders would tackle the practical implications of these threats, the RRF was tasked with monitoring more intangible signs of system-wide groundswells of public concern, reactions, and debates: issues which are too vast and remote to belong within crisis leaders' own field of vision, but which the RRF ensures do not go overlooked either. Loss of telephone systems, as noted above, would especially "inject huge energy into the crisis," and compound every other issue, while also cementing unrelated disruptions into a single overarching crisis: as it would not only undermine awareness, but also reduce all stakeholders' field of vision to their individual, emotional concern for the welfare of loved ones.

Interestingly, this shortlist was the subject of considerable debate among our participants, reflecting cultural differences in risk assessment among countries. Most notably, American colleagues tended to believe that the public would be most preoccupied with the single suicide bombing incident on U.S. soil that our scenario premised; while others argued that the pandemic threat would remain front and center among people's concerns, and was a more pressing priority in the allocation of responders' limited time and resources.

Critical pitfalls

In addition to prioritizing challenges, crisis responders in our exercise were also careful to *remain in control of linkage among issues*; as such linkage would determine the general architecture of response mechanisms, so would hold crucial implications for responders' margin of maneuver. In particular, the "leadership group" among our participants decided against spending time to explore whether emerging diseases had in fact been caused by Islamic terrorists, in spite of the existence (and visibility) of al-Qaeda threats. This potential linkage was deemed only to hold "over the horizon" implications, as it might shift public perceptions of the crisis if it came to be confirmed; yet for the time being, crisis leaders realized that their decision-making process would remain mostly identical in either case, and chose to task the RRF with monitoring the issue rather than letting it tinge or crowd their own radar screen. As a participant put it, "The al-Qaeda threat is there, we're aware of it: but *we're not going to let it 'manage' us* or drive us right now."

While leadership might eschew artificial and unhelpful linkages, there is no guarantee that all other stakeholders would do so as well. They might instead create *"stigmatizing linkages"* that would single out a community for suspicion and blame, thus shifting and poisoning the debate, undermining cohesion and trust among responders and the greater public, and providing interstices in which the crisis would thrive. A participant, for instance, looked at our scenario through this prism, specifically at the al-Qaeda threat, and at the premise that communicable diseases had broken out in Muslim countries and among Muslim populations elsewhere.

> "The question is whether or not *somebody* somewhere will say: 'it's something about *that* particular group.' We might then see NGOs jumping up and down about human rights in defense of this population. It seems to me that one of the things that always happens is this contest between trying to embrace all people and say 'we're all part of the same problem,' but also at the same time, people looking for culpability, looking for easy answers. And that divisiveness, it seems to me, is really one of the big issues."

One apparent—but self-defeating—way out of the complexity of our scenario would be to eschew *any linkage* whatsoever among issues, a process driven less by a conscious decision to do so than by internal dynamics of bureaucratic silos within each country, as each would simply go about tackling the facet of the problem that belonged in its remit. In our exercise, the "Rapid Reflection Force" group set out to counteract the pull of this cultural comfort zone. As a participant explained, "The first thing is that we recognized that this is a multinational, system-wide combination of events. And that, therefore, it did not make sense for decision-making to be based on single jurisdiction-interests and single-jurisdiction policies."

The danger inherent in self-absorbed silos would especially be heightened in our scenario, as they would all remain blind to the fact that the multiplicity of simultaneous disruptions might well reach a "critical mass" leading to the unthinkable collapse of existing systemic architecture and social compacts. Here we enter the *terra incognita* of brewing revolutions; this is a terrain which crisis leaders certainly cannot explore themselves, but which underlines the value of RRFstyle unconventional crisis cells whose field of vision is vast enough to encompass such looming threats. It is indeed not beyond the realm of the possible that our globalized societies, past a critical threshold in "systemic shocks," would suddenly put in question basic value systems and political processes, such as underlie the legitimacy and power of crisis response leaders in the first place. Daring to look at this contingency is not the stuff of naïve Cassandras; just as a Charles I in 1648, a Louis XVI in 1788 would have been well advised to acknowledge that the systems they ruled might come to fall, with their head.

Our scenario itself included the proposition that the International Federation of the Red Cross in Geneva would call a summit of NGOs to coordinate their response to the very large number of flu victims that were forecast in the circumstances; and that they would conclude their meeting with a scathing indictment of governments' performance, suggesting that they might well take matters into their own hands. Going one step further, our "red team" looked most earnestly at the notion that an "unthinkable" coalition of civil society representatives, in the face of so many threats, and feeding on public fear, uncertainty, and loss of trust, might proclaim that "the world as we know it has ceased to exist." As a participant eloquently explained,

> "While we should tackle the issues that are clearly out there, I believe that we also should open a file marked: 'unknown.' Face the blank page. Because as soon as the 'page is written over,' tunnel vision kicks in.
> So the question is: is there an overall, global challenge at hand here? The crucial watershed of emerging crises occurs when you move from *difficulties*, to a *vacuum*. For instance, we could see a global perception of *loss of control*, which could trigger inconceivable domino effects, massive disruptions, sky-rocketing anxiety—including among leaders themselves! And this huge anxiety rapidly would produce bunker effects, so that it would become very difficult to work across stovepipes. If this impression takes hold, it would undermine the entire system that's been in place: 'we thought leaders were controlling the world, but it turns out nobody is in control of anything any more.' And it would have a terrible effect on the system's balance.

So I would open another line of questioning, I would dare to open this 'unknown,' blank page. And I think that we still very much have to learn how to navigate these strange environments: crises outside the box."

Mapping partners and spoilers

Participants taking the mantle of government leaders in our exercise exhibited a keen sense that other stakeholders would be critical to response efforts—most notably private industry, NGOs, and the media. Though this by itself might well be an improvement on traditional public sector assumptions, it did not entirely avoid problematic cultural bents, most notably the notion that these "partners" could be "brought in" and be "coordinated" by government so that the latter could "tap into" their resources and expertise.

This, however, failed to take account of the looming uncertainty whether such partners would agree to be *coordinated* by government, or in fact by *anyone*. It seemed doubtful that international NGOs would be much impressed by governments' draping themselves in the cloak of "sovereignty." The same issue arose most clearly in the case of public sector efforts to "get the media on board." Some participants suggested that government, in their own country at least, would certainly have no sway whatsoever on editorial decisions—and highlighted that, in any case, the increasingly dominant blogosphere simply was too complex and independent to engage in any sort of structured dialogue with public sector leadership, let alone cooperate with it. A colleague tied the two issues together, arguing that in most Western countries, when faced with catastrophic events, "traditional media *will* play along initially: but the amount of time they'll do so is affected by the behavior of the new media. Once the alternative sources come forward, the mainstream media will also break ranks, as they can't see their credibility fall flat."

An equally problematic coalition that might be needed based on our scenario would combine health systems and the military. A participant underlined that "due to the lack of surge capacity in public health systems, military assistance through field hospitals might be required in a major pandemic." In this case again serious doubt would exist regarding the ability of both parties culturally to avoid a dialogue of the deaf, and organizationally to agree on a decision-making hierarchy; while the public's response to such a contingency also would be a matter for concern. As the same colleague was quick to add, "responders would have to prepare the public to something that looked like the response to the 1918 Spanish flu."

Faced with our scenario, participants in the "red team" quickly identified the most powerful potential spoilers: voices that would emerge from the nebulous worlds of traditional or "new" media (now including Twitter) to shape collective understanding of the challenges at hand, most notably by drawing linkages among issues, or exaggerating the resulting threats, irrespective of the evidence. "What type of propaganda would be out there, trying to heighten that level of fear and mistrust?" New messages from al-Qaeda explicitly claiming responsibility for the outbreak of communicable diseases would of course be the most spectacular factor in shaping global perceptions; but equally deleterious, though less visible among threats lurking beyond the horizon, would be the "thousand cuts" of innumerable opinions driving the debate so far from the facts that crisis responders would find themselves out of touch with the greater public.

The variety of international stakeholders involved in our scenario would also produce an explosive overlap between response efforts and subjacent geopolitical conflicts—a risk clearly underlined by the premise that a clash would recur between Gazprom and Ukraine. Thus, our "red team" highlighted the potential consequences of a state of play where, in the face of a pandemic, developed nations would hold medical assets (such as masks and vaccine supplies), while developing countries symmetrically would retain control of the former's lifeblood, especially in the form of energy resources; potentially causing a critical "face-off" where the latter would utilize their leverage in order to access medical equipment.

Spoilers and vicious circles, however, need not be so sinister or apocalyptic. Again, the most pressing threat is one of cumulated, though individually minute impacts—the risk that, in the absence of reliable information, elements in the response system will "break rank," lose their defensive shape along with their nerve, and resort to "knee-jerk reactions" in order to save themselves, or simply to "do something."

This danger, then, ultimately ties into the broader issue of crisis communication strategies from upper-tier leadership.

Critical initiatives

Considerable experience with ill-thought outreach efforts informs our participants' views on crisis communication. As we have seen, they argue that leaders faced with "unthinkable" disruptions should not—which they often do—fall under the illusion that they can only uphold their legitimacy and prevent panic if they present a "united front of omniscience" when speaking out to the public. This approach holds the potential for catastrophic breakdowns of trust, once the veil is lifted on the extent of leaders' ignorance—as it soon must be. In addition, it causes responders to delay public pronouncements until they "have collected all the facts," and thus to speak out too late, once their deafening silence already has caused the emergence of more relevant and trusted voices.

The purpose of crisis communication is not, then, to reassert leaders' superior awareness of all facts; only they believe this to be the source of their legitimacy. Continued demonstration of their omniscience might be what leaders culturally expect of themselves in crisis situations, but not so the public; partial ignorance is not the weak point in leaders' legitimacy, not the interstice into which the crisis will thrive. Instead, leaders must reassure their constituents that *responders still retain the initiative*, that a sound decision-making process is alive and well, that the ship of state is not rudderless; and that its course is intelligible, albeit based on imperfect information. As a participant explained when reacting to our scenario,

> "Very rapidly the leader would be out in front of the media, saying: 'This is how we've organized ourselves, this is what we're doing. *We don't know* if there are links or not between disease breakouts and terrorism, but we'll carry on. We've established these committees; this is how we're beginning to approach the problems.'"

The need for a cultural shift in the motivations and objectives of crisis communication was further highlighted by a participant who argued that crisis leaders responding to our scenario should have consulted the "red team" before speaking out to the public, in order to ensure that they would not "get the *really* bad news *after* they had been in front of the media."

Of course, our exercise assumed that physical infrastructure underlying mass communications had itself been impacted. The RRF group quickly flagged this challenge as a "hub" in the "structure of crisis," since mitigating the problem could go a long way towards resolving several issues at once. Thus our unconventional crisis cell—reflecting the value-added of its unusual make-up, which combines strategists and technical experts—set to work on identifying workarounds for disrupted communication systems.

In addition to restoring these capabilities, the RRF team also focused on a critical challenge which we highlighted above: recovering control over *time*. In the face of unrelenting pressure on the international financial system, our participants recommended a "reset" in the "chronology of crisis" by calling upon crisis leaders to initiate a prolonged bank holiday: aiming "to reestablish IT systems that had been damaged, rethink strategies within the banking sector, and—perhaps more importantly than either of those—to restore confidence within the general public."

Consistent with their remit, then, the RRF and red teams approached the scenario from a different standpoint than the "leadership team," and did provide the latter with unconventional proposals. Yet instances when their respective thought process and radar screen converged by no means undermined the value-added of these mechanisms. On the contrary, this overlap recreated an *"intelligent comfort zone"* in the face of the unconventional, which was all the more precious as leadership was called upon to take "critical initiatives" that would have remained angst-inducing leaps of faith without some reassurance that unconventional crisis cells had reached identical conclusions. As a participant from the RRF team noted when addressing the leadership group, "even when we were suggesting things to you that you were already thinking yourself, while it may not have added substance to what you were doing, it added a level of comfort that perhaps you were on the right track."

Leadership structures should not be left in a splendid isolation when making critical decisions with imperfect information—whether this isolation is self-imposed, the result of leaders' ill-advised belief in their own omniscience, or derives from other stakeholders' self-serving wish to wash their hands of such decisions and let leaders alone sink with the ship if they make the wrong call. A colleague noted that in too many exercises or real-life situations, a leader's performance in unconventional environments becomes "a reflection on their entire character; the notion being that 'you're really good at it, or you're not.'" Rather than conjuring heroic figures—also "villains" or "incompetent frauds" when facing unconventional crises (9/11's Rudy Giuliani and Katrina's Michael Brown respectively come to mind), organizations and public opinion should realize that the quality of response will rather depend on intelligent structures that will support leadership in chaotic environments.

Redrawing Cross-Sector Allocations of Tasks

Certainly there is nothing new in advocating a more effective "public-private partnership," and our project's participants are under no illusion that simply repeating the mantra would allow them to break new ground. More to the point, the same mantra, by itself, badly fails to meet the challenges at hand. Recent events have heightened the sense of urgency in bringing about more effective cross-silo cooperation, as they have highlighted the considerable price to be paid when impediments prevent or undermine it. Based proximately on an examination of the risks involved in global pandemics and other public health contingencies, we set to work, then, on more innovative analyses of cross-sector relationships.

Public sector perspectives

Building cross-sector fields of vision

Our 2008 report began with a taxonomy of crises that included "insidious events." It is important, however, to realize that a disruption is never "insidious" *per se*, but only because the structure of responders' fields of vision *makes it so*. Absent a "grand bargain" among sectors that would build up a combined, intelligent radar screen, each silo's specific blind spot remains unchallenged, and indeed threatens to contaminate other sectors' own field of vision—thus creating, and compounding, insidious disruptions. This unfortunately is the situation that still prevails today in public-sector epidemiology, where a "splendid isolation" among government officials and public health experts undermines their ability to flag complex disruptions. As one of our participants put it, "most of the risks that we confront today are what I term 'invisible risks': meaning that no single stakeholder can observe them—and specifically that doctors in their hospitals, or officials in cabinet ministries, cannot see them."

This means that such events will be left to simmer until they spectacularly shed their "insidious" nature, and become observable on radar screens, once they turn into catastrophic crises: once it is *too late*.

At the interface between leadership culture and behavior, a cascade of mental blocks and delayed action reflects the problem—which much transcends the specific case of epidemiology.

- First: government *is blind* to the existence of public health risks.

- Second: it *hears about emerging warning signals* from *other sources*, but it denies that a problem truly exists.

- Third: warning signals accumulate, but government does not act upon them.

- Fourth, government acknowledges the problem, but plays it down.

- Fifth, government finally reacts, but is poorly prepared, and has lost control over the pace of the crisis by waiting too long.

Nor is public sector alone in exhibiting such symptoms. In fact, the same participant best illustrated the poverty of silo-specific fields of vision when he quoted an illuminating conversation between the head of a private sector chemical company, and a journalist pressing him on the apparent carcinogenic effects of one of his products. Digging an ever deeper hole for himself, the interviewee explained in all seriousness, for instance, that "there is no definite proof that our product may cause cancer. *Internally*, we have never seen any conclusive sign that it does. *Our best guess*, if I may put it that way, is that there is no unusual occurrence of cancer in our profession."

The 2003 heat wave in Europe provides a telling example of a challenge which remained insidious in the absence of cross-silo radar screens. As we explained above, it was so shocking and so challenging because the battlefield, and the matrix of the problem, was not truly hospitals' ERs, and their lack of surge capacity, but rather communities throughout Western Europe, towns and villages, residential buildings and houses' attics—isolated seniors who were looked after by no one. Conventional conduits that typically fed bottom-up information into government's field of vision were therefore inadequate, as the most relevant "observers" were neither hospitals nor regional authorities, but a disjointed mosaic of families, neighbors, and local social services.

In the wake of the crisis, then, France built up a more diverse and multi-layered early warning system to collect epidemiological data from a broader spectrum of sources, thus creating a multi-focal, intelligent field of vision. More broadly, a participant argued that

> "Cross-sector early warning and monitoring systems today are essential to confront unconventional crises. Because when you build up such a system, you create a framework that will organize public debate; help make sense of the threat; and prod stakeholders who had never worked with one another to sit at the same table, before a crisis hits. In addition, it promotes a culture where stakeholders will focus on collecting facts, rather than indulging in clashes of individual opinions. Third, these mechanisms make it possible to agree ahead of time upon a common definition of what 'alert thresholds' will be. Lastly, they can be used for joint assessments of response efforts once a crisis has subsided."

Cross-silo response efforts

Just as the 2003 heat wave remained insidious and elusive in the absence of a combined field of vision, effective response would have required cross-silo mechanisms. Since all sectors of society, to include the greater public, were guilty parties in the crisis, only a joint response effort could have prevented or mitigated it. Cutting through silos, however, has remained a daunting challenge, due to organizational as well as cultural obstacles.

Thus, in most instances, governments' initial plans to confront flu pandemics took little if any account of private industry, other than pharmaceutical companies. Meanwhile, most private sector leaders used to dismiss the threat as one that only concerned public health systems, and had little import for their companies. Certainly, much progress has since been made on both counts, not least because actual pandemics have awoken all stakeholders to the nature of the challenge. Yet much remains to be done.

Most notably, the evidence suggests that a cultural bent still prevails among certain strata of governments against being fully forthcoming as to the contents of pandemic plans—based on the fear that they might, for instance, disclose military assets and planning, to include force protection. This temptation to superimpose a culture of secrecy upon homeland security planning certainly is not specific to any country in particular, though it has manifested itself more acutely in some of them. It has been especially problematic when governments have chosen to classify an *entire* plan, rather than its most sensitive sections. As a participant lamented, "Personally, I'm not sure what to do with a plan that requires coordinated efforts from all sectors, yet is classified so cannot be shared with any outside stakeholder..." Indeed such roadblocks have resulted in private companies, for instance, being unable to produce workable pandemic plans, at least such as would ensure effective coordination with the public sector.

Governments' reluctance to be more forthcoming on matters of homeland security is merely an example of a broader cultural obstacle that we noted above: namely, the public sector's traditional assumption that "building a large tent" means inviting outside partners to join in an effort whose strategic direction will remain *exclusively* in the hands of government—thus limiting their contribution to "filling the occasional gap" in public sector response or assets. Epidemiological threats shed an interesting light on the problem, as ultimate responsibility for system-wide efforts and societal mobilization to confront such risks certainly must lie with elected officials, while at the same time the proposition that they hold the only, or even the most important assets for response is often mistaken. As a participant underlined,

> "Some private companies today have become more powerful than states. So have certain NGOs. Today, the most powerful figure in the public health field, without any doubt, is Bill Gates. The budget of his foundation is ten times larger than that of the WHO. The ratio of scales has entirely shifted away from the public sector."

Preventing "orphan crises"

Cutting through silos in preparing for and responding to crisis is especially important because failing to do so will create *orphan crises*, and therefore let otherwise mundane disruptions slide into the "unthinkable." As a participant explained, "our world brings about situations in which no one is answerable for risks."

Some applications of nanotechnology illustrate the point. Certain companies have been adding nanometric traces of titanium dioxide in the cement they produce. This substance is harmless, *except* at a nanometric scale, when it has recently been shown to hold risks for human genetic material. Faced with this problem, cement companies can argue that they simply buy titanium dioxide from others, and thus cannot be responsible, as "they weren't told that there was a problem"; while the source of the incriminated product will explain that they did not sell it in toxic nanometric quantities, so are equally free of blame.

The complexity of commercial relationships today threatens to produce exponential numbers of such "orphan crises," as each silo evaluates risk and acts upon it based on its own radar screen, its specific remit, and its narrowly defined regulatory environment. The problem arises not only across sectors, but within them, as each building block replicates the same inward-looking approach, and therefore dissolves answerability. This explains a participant's remark that "within government, I am no longer clear as to who leads my department. Ministers are disconnected from their own administration; they work with the media, with elected officials in parliament, rather than with their own civil servants."

Responsibility has been broken asunder. When this mosaic does not simply dilute accountability altogether, it leads to politically motivated, facile, or simply random "surges of finger-pointing," as coalescing narratives suddenly lay *all* the blame at the feet of one among countless other responsible parties, whether politicians, the media, private industry, NGOs, etc.

Finding a solution to this problem entails the creation of "partnerships of responsibility" that will be as complex as the crises they confront, and thus enable the "reemergence of accountability." This objective, however, remains all the more elusive as individual stakeholders can be tempted to turn the "limbos of responsibility" into a momentarily reassuring, though ultimately suicidal comfort zone.

Views from other sectors

Calling on government to do its job

Throughout the present report we consistently call for government to realize that it must facilitate others' efforts, rather than stifle them by entertaining the mistaken belief that it holds a monopoly on all aspects of decision-making in crisis situations. This does certainly not imply, however, that government should be deprived of all leadership—quite the contrary, as being an effective "facilitator" has considerable implications. Though government must learn to share responsibility and initiative with other stakeholders in a vast swath of the strategic and operational field, it retains a monopoly on paramount decisions that only it can take, "upstream" of both dimensions: namely in establishing a legislative and regulatory framework, and nurturing a collective sense of purpose and direction.

This, however, it sometimes fails to achieve. As a participant lamented when drawing the lessons of the SARS outbreak,

> "There's an enormous reluctance on the part of governments to make fundamental decisions: governments don't want to commit to who's going to lead; they don't want to commit to what our mask policy is going to be; or to how big the anti-viral supply will be, and whether it will be used for prevention, treatment, or post-exposure prophylaxis. And I don't know *how* you establish a proper plan if you haven't made a decision on such fundamental questions. Governments don't want to lay out the implications of a pandemic, they don't want to say who's going to be protected in what way. Everybody knows what the policies should be: but nobody wants to commit to them publicly. Governments seem to be satisfied that they'll solve the problem by just ignoring it. Well, all we'll have then is chaos."

Certainly one of the impediments that has deterred the public sector from tackling such questions more forcefully has been the political cost to pay for triggering suspicions of "government's overreaching"—or more sinister yet, of government "utilizing the crisis as an opportunity to expand its control over people's lives." The truth is, however, that unconventional crises hold such system-wide implications that they *will* pose tough questions of social compacts and political culture; the only choice at hand, then, is whether political leaders and the public alike can muster the vision and will to have the inevitable debate *before* such a crisis hits, or in the midst of it, when the dangers of overreach surely are most acute.

Understanding the private sector

Thus, failing to take its responsibilities in making fundamental decisions that will create an intelligible framework for response, government impedes the efforts of other sectors by leaving them to navigate a blurred battlefield on their own. In addition, however, it often restrains their margin of maneuver, or issues unrealistic demands, based on a faulty understanding of other stakeholders' motives and priorities. A participant argued the point when discussing port and maritime security:

> "There is a belief prevalent in parts of the government that somehow they can tell business how to get their cargoes into the United States in case of an emergency: 'we will direct them to this port or that port, and we will tell them which trains to use,' etc. In fact, they won't have a thing to say about it! They may close or open ports; but shipping companies will rebuild their strategy based on their own self-interest, because their lifeblood is delivering cargo to customers; and they'll find a way to get it over the border and in to their customers *without government.* So I think government needs to think very hard about what it *doesn't know* with regard to private industry. Government doesn't understand business very well—in any country."

The irrelevance of public sector suspicion

This lack of understanding has manifested itself most notably in government's tendency to ascribe private industry's efforts in crisis response exclusively to the pursuit of profit—or indeed to outright gouging. This pervasive suspicion, in fact, has been a permanent impediment to progress on cross-sector cooperation, both in planning and, regrettably, in actual response efforts. However, it suffers from two fundamental problems.

First, though it does reflect incentive structures that undeniably spur private industry, this interpretation partakes in a popular caricature and blanket indictment which government should eschew, or at least refine, if only out of concern for the effectiveness of crisis response. As we shall see below, the private sector has demonstrated time and again that ethical considerations could in fact weigh upon its own decision-making, as could a sense of responsibility *vis-à-vis* local communities of employees and clients: not indeed *aside* from profit motives, but because major crises turn the welfare of local communities into *the ultimate implication and precondition of sustainable profit seeking.*

Yet, in a larger sense, the nature of private industry's motives is irrelevant. The proposition that government should be suspicious of them implies the illusion that, when faced with unconventional crises, the public sector will somehow have the *luxury* of double-guessing the private sector's ethics, or indeed anyone else's; that it will have a choice whether or not to *bring* private industry *into* response efforts, based on an appreciation of its incentives. The truth is that private industry *will already be there*, indeed at the forefront of defensive lines, among the victims, permeating the entire response environment, critical to all response efforts—much before government even *recovers its own relevance*. This, indeed, is the paramount implication of the oft-repeated fact that private industry, in the U.S., "owns 85 percent of critical infrastructure."

New social compact vs. government withdrawal

A (belated) realization that the private sector will play such a decisive role in unconventional crises, combined with "post-traumatic" concern among governmental officials that they incur excessive political cost from repeated failures to live up to culturally embedded expectations as to government's effectiveness, has in fact led the public sector to reconsider cross-sector allocations of tasks.

However, this evolution potentially holds a critical danger, reflecting the stark differences in the implications of these two motivations. Calling on private sector and NGOs to take on more responsibilities in the response to unconventional crises is unhelpful if it simply means that government withdraws from the field and relinquishes its fundamental responsibilities in the face of such threats, in the process leaving other sectors with ill-defined remits that much exceed their comfort zone, expertise, and legal liability.

In 2008, as in 2007, a number of participants from private industry recalled their dismay when told by the U.S. government, in the wake of Katrina, that they would henceforth be expected to assume a more prominent role in crisis response—though deprived of the legal and strategic guidelines, or operational assets, that would enable them to meet the challenge. This amounted—perilously—to government simply throwing the towel and disengaging from the fight: as a mistaken and bloated understanding of public sector leadership had led it to a symmetrically excessive reaction in concluding that it should pass the baton to other players.

> "The question begs itself: what are we responsible for, in the private sector? The government's call for corporations to 'take more responsibility for citizens' has put us in a difficult position: because it is not clearly defined. What does it mean? Does it mean that we're responsible for our staff? What about their extended families? Where do we draw the line? How do we make the decision on who goes home, and who doesn't? And all the while, private sector and NGOs are kept at arm's length from decision-making, and often aren't even allowed to enter the impacted zone. So we as corporate crisis managers would want to have a clearer vision of our level of responsibility."

Redrawing allocations of tasks among sectors, and across levels of governance (from local to international) is welcome if prodded by a realistic assessment of the decisive input of non-governmental stakeholders, but lethal if driven by government's illusion that it can simply disengage. Efforts to redefine cross-sector responsibilities, then, will be doomed if not based on preliminary clarification of the political and strategic considerations that motivate the process in the first place.

The "right reasons" behind the renegotiation of a cross-silo "social compact" are easy enough to grasp: they lie in the realization that hyper-complex events will distribute leadership, and prod its emergence from unconventional sources, irrespective of organization charts, through all sectors and strata: so that governments, private sector, NGOs and civil society must establish *a priori* guidelines that will ensure that this redistribution is not entirely imposed upon them by crisis, or seen as an unthinkable development that will paralyze response systems and instantly undermine preexisting plans.

The solution must come from government finally desisting from superimposing national security culture and models upon homeland security (which in part entails that it turn away from excessive focaliza-tion on terrorism at the expense of other threats): in other words, relin-quishing top-down, single-chain of command structures, and the cul-ture of secrecy, in order to leverage the subjacent strength that lies in concerted dialogue and initiatives among civil society broadly defined.

Others, most notably Stephen Flynn, have long been clamoring for such a cultural change, and have provided insightful and detailed guid-ance on how to effect it. Our participants emphatically seconded the point: advocating a denser web of "civil society relationships," based upon sustained strategic dialogue, operational coordination, and a clearer allocation of tasks among public and private sector, as well as not-for-profit groups, faith-based organizations, foundations, local communities' representatives, even influential individuals. While this framework would nurture local initiatives and local ownership of risk and needs assessment, turning government into their "enabler," partic-ipants also recommended that agreements be reached in advance upon "red lines" that would trigger a switch from a "pull" to a "push" system past a certain degree in the seriousness of crises—thus ensuring that the cultivation of bottom-up, inclusive dynamics does not turn into a structural weakness.

Certainly, then, a new social compact is needed to confront uncon-ventional crises—yet one that will reflect not government's *dis*engage-ment, but a "new birth" of its engagement with other sectors, based upon revised cultural foundations.

Enhancing Systemic Resiliency

As we highlighted in our 2008 report, unconventional events do not simply create localized wounds in systems—do not simply impact a "ground zero" surrounded by an "unscathed outside"—but produce systemic shocks, for two reasons: first because they affect complex, interdependent networks, or "superstructures," that are only as resilient as their weakest link, or node; and second because they cause a *sepsis* of the lifeblood that flows within these superstructures. As a participant explained, resiliency can only be ensured if organizations take into account "structural interdependence among various industries; but also the human factor: men and women who will enable the system to go on, or prevent it from doing so. And if we only make progress on one of the two issues, we will have made no progress at all."

In the face of these system-wide impacts, resiliency must be *deep*, it must be *adaptive*, and it must be *holistic*. In other words, it cannot simply be the preserve of a lone agency within each organization specialized in putting out fires, digging trenches, or "quarantining" affected limbs to ensure "business continuity"; nor can it stem from the paradigm that everything can be protected against all hazards by drawing static defense lines. Finally, it cannot be a mere addendum, an afterthought, a "segment" restricted in time and remit to a clearly defined "post-crisis phase": on the contrary, efforts towards resiliency must permeate the entire "chronology" of organizations, from the moment their architecture is defined, transcending the chasm between "peace time" and "crisis time."

Structural resiliency

Unconventional events such as 9/11 and Katrina have gone a long way towards convincing stakeholders of the need to take pragmatic measures in order to reinforce their critical networks, through duplication, diversification, or geographical diffusion.

After the attacks on the World Trade Center brought critical infrastructure to the brim of collapse, or indeed past it, the Federal Reserve Bank, the Securities Exchange Commission, and the Department of

Treasury joined forces to publish an *Interagency Paper on Sound Practices to Strengthen the Resilience of the U.S. Financial System*. Based on the definition of three different tiers among financial organizations, reflecting their respective importance as critical links or nodes within the industry, the paper especially mandated companies that carried vital systemic risk to develop a resilient footprint by diversifying both their technical and human resources out of Manhattan. Technical centers and workforce were relocated e.g. into upstate New York, Canada, the Midwest, or Florida (in the latter case arguably exchanging one set of risks for another). This new geography entailed structural and human resources challenges, but most importantly a cultural revolution, as the move out of New York City went against the grain of gregarious centralization in the industry.

Superstructure resiliency

Such efforts to reinforce structural resiliency within a particular industry (or a particular Emergency Support Function, in an American context) are laudable, but insufficient. Indeed they still reflect the narrow field of vision of bureaucratic silos, which go about taking action within their specific remit without taking account of their dependency on other sectors—or doubting that they could in fact coordinate their efforts with any one else's in an effective manner. However, 9/11 itself abundantly made clear that the financial sector's best efforts to diversify and relocate its critical assets would achieve nothing if undertaken in isolation from other critical infrastructure, such as telecommunications, whose paralysis or collapse would trigger cross-industry domino effects. "Organizations can focus on their own sector; or their own supply chain; but unconventional events involve *everyone*: governments, first responders, the private sector...: everyone. And if any one of those links breaks along that chain, all of a sudden you become vulnerable."

Thus, when France was hit by two hurricane-strength storms within a week at the end of 1999, delays in the restoration of the electrical grid pulled the rug from under the feet of every other infrastructure provider. "Within three days, telecommunication companies were impacted because cell phone batteries had run out; after four or five days, sewage and water treatment companies were down; while transportation systems, most notably electricity-powered trains, were also paralyzed."

Faced with this interdependency, a solution was highlighted by a number of participants: namely setting up an international forum, a "network of networks" among critical infrastructure providers, upstream of crisis, *if only* so they can know one another, and start mapping out the issues—much transcending the ESF format both in terms of the depth of thinking, and the geographical scope of the effort. Uniquely in the face of unconventional events, the identity of relevant stakeholders is clear: the challenge is not to determine who should sit at the table, but how to bring them there in the first place.

Certainly the U.S. (among others) in recent years has woken up to the need to create inter-sector and inter-industry roundtables ahead of crises. This is most evident in a number of ambitious exercises that have combined a broad spectrum of stakeholders, with an international dimension—and therefore have much improved upon the 2004 "Hurricane Pam" model, which infamously kept private industry at the door. We are on our way, and moving in the right direction; but the destination is still remote, and we must quicken our pace.

Obstacles remain in the underlying culture of the public sector, which still sees itself as the self-evident leader of "*public-private*" exercises, kindly inviting outsiders into governmental situation rooms. This fails to reflect not only the preeminent role that private industry *will* play in unconventional crises: but also, most often, the increasingly powerful and independent realm of non-governmental organizations, whose numbers have mushroomed with their financial resources, and which now exert considerable influence over international *norms*, while also commanding unmatched legitimacy and trust from the greater public. Impediments also arise from the motivation of private-sector participants in these training drills, as competitors might use these occasions to access restricted information or otherwise undermine the preeminence of industry leaders. In addition, government has been reluctant to send upper-tier leadership to the table, preferring to dispatch mid-level civil servants who would not in fact hold the levers of power in unconventional crises. Most critically, of course, these exercises share in the fatal weakness that we identified above—they typically aim for the symbolic reassertion of existing power structures and legitimacy, through the validation of static bodies of knowledge, and therefore exhibit considerable reluctance to anticipate unconventional contingencies.

Lifeblood resiliency: the human dimension

"Do not lose your vital human assets." Unconventional crises have proved that there is more to this precept—at least if understood intelligently—than a facile business-school mantra. Restoring structure-specific and superstructure capabilities is useless if it results in a system whose arteries run fine but whose blood cells are sick. "You can have the best footprint and systems in terms of infrastructure: but if you lose your people, all you'll be left with is a beautiful tool and no one to use it."

The challenge in this multi-pronged approach to resiliency is that while structural and superstructure improvements result from top-down architectural planning, ensuring the resiliency of "lifeblood" can only be achieved through bottom-up dynamics. As a participant explained when discussing the avian flu,

> "Our company and our industry were mandated to work from a plan that had been prepared by government, focusing on business continuity. But as we set out to do so, we faced a critical obstacle: as, by definition, we could not know in advance how many employees could be counted on to implement the plan in case of a pandemic. So we had to rethink the problem 'upside down': and leave the initiative to each business unit manager on the ground so they could find flexible ways to work things out based on the workforce that would be available to them, finding *ad hoc* replacement for sick or missing employees."

Such bottom-up approaches can only tap into and organize underlying collective strength that will enable populations to pull through unconventional events. These resources, to an extent, depend upon the capacity of upper-tier leadership to produce a common sense of purpose, and a horizon of hope; yet at bottom they reflect the inherent "spine" and fortitude of populations. As our participants underlined, system-wide unconventional disruptions can only be confronted through equally broad mobilization, i.e. a more or less intangible *"community spirit."*

Therein, indeed, lies a fundamental challenge in unconventional crises. While "normal" disruptions can be met through static lines of defense at the margins of systems, acute and hypercomplex crises will ask fundamental questions of populations' solidarity, courage, and self-reliance. A participant noted, however, that sixty years of peace have placed a question mark over the cultural capacity of European populations to confront "unthinkable" disruptions: an avatar of Robert Kagan's indictment of "Kantian Europe," and one of the most critical consequences of the continent's alleged wallowing in the illusions of perpetual peace and unshakable safety—both of which the public believes are ensured by leaders who will be omniscient and omnipotent in the face of crisis, will restore systemic normalcy in an instant, or else "come to the rescue within 72 hours." Though the diagnosis that the West, and Europe in particular, have "lost their spine" is debatable, and must remain a hypothetical proposition until tested by events, what is not in question is that "stiff upper lips" are a cultivated habit, rather than a matter of innate stoicism granted by providence upon chosen people—and that the habit has *not* been cultivated in the recent history of the West. If this remains the case, bottom-up dynamics aiming to channel "lifeblood resiliency" will find no underlying strength to tap into and mobilize.

In any event, the bottom-up character of human resiliency does not exempt upper-tier leadership from undertaking a strategic effort to *map out* predictable drivers that will affect human behavior when unconventional crises hit. Relevant factors on this "map" are numerous, but clear: a shortlist would include people's health, their concern for loved ones, bottlenecks in underlying systems such as transportation, and sundry human passions such as loss of trust, fear, and—rarely—outright panic.

This "mapping" effort, however, can only be successful if based on the paradigm that the resiliency of the "human lifeblood" is no more silo-specific than that of structural, technical assets. In other words, organizations' ability to sustain unconventional crises will not only be affected by the welfare of their own employees: but by that of their clients as well, and indeed by dynamics that will permeate the entire human environment in which they operate. Thus, following Katrina, private companies suddenly came to realize that they had become their "brothers' keepers," unlikely champions of neighboring communities, which called upon them to transcend *normal* profit incentives in their decision-making. Though their initiatives in this respect were often driven by ethical considerations, there was more (and less) to the efforts of Wal-Mart, Accor, Home Depot and others than just good will and a sense of neighborly solidarity: as these measures ultimately were a prerequisite for their own survival through the crisis (or at least that of their local branches). Thus,

> "When the head of a local New Orleans bank arrived in Houston after he had evacuated the city, and was told by a hotel clerk that his credit card had been refused and that he 'didn't exist in the system,' he realized that if that was true in his case, then there were millions of people out there, clients or neighbors of his, who 'didn't exist in the system' either; and that his mission had changed. He understood that his task in Houston wasn't simply to organize his company's backup mechanisms, but to follow up with impacted populations, to set up cash-only systems, to assist them through the crisis and help people *resist*."

In other words, resiliency properly understood transcends the preservation of infrastructure or employees' know-how; it also depends upon defense mechanisms that will sustain one's *core business* in the broadest sense of the term, to include private industry's responsibility *vis-à-vis* local populations. Again, this is not only a matter of ethics, of "going the extra mile"—it is certainly not a matter of "looking good" or "burnishing one's brand." It is part and parcel of sustainability and survival, including very pragmatic financial considerations. Thus the New Orleans bank mentioned above "achieved the best bottom line among its competitors one year after the storm. Why? Because its clients *trusted* it; they never lost confidence in this bank."

Distributed leadership

Structural and superstructure resiliency will especially benefit from human fortitude if the emergence of unanticipated sources of leadership—which, as we have seen, is a defining feature of unconventional crises—is funneled into culturally prevalent, strategically sound, and operationally actionable dynamics, rather than being seen as an intolerable impediment for the implementation of overly static plans. This implies spreading leadership throughout defensive systems, which in turn will prevent "single point of failure" vulnerability.

Doing so, indeed, can "turn the tables" on unconventional crises. While they thrive on an organization's blind zones, the organization can return the favor by also exploiting *the blind zones of crisis*, which always exist if one would only look for them. Such events, like a Great Flood, will leave metaphorical "Ararat mountaintops" unscathed; the challenge is to set up leadership structures that can lay claim to this safe ground, in order to regroup and organize the counter-attack. The first such mechanism is simply to multiply the actors that can potentially do so within the organization: in other words, to "spread out" leadership; which, in concrete terms, implies that employees be dual-hatted throughout, and be trained as crisis leaders in addition to their "peace time" job.

Some of the private companies that performed best through Katrina, for instance, had set up a dual allocation of responsibility, and chain of command, respectively for "peace time" and "crisis time," based upon employees' underlying crisis-management skills, which were continually nurtured through training drills, and benefited from a corporate culture that accepted the instant reshaping of hierarchical structure when crisis struck.

This suggests that organizations should imbed within their architecture the capacity to switch habits and mechanisms from the "normal" to the "unconventional mode," by assuming "twin identities" and cultures throughout the system, reflecting both types of challenges—which presupposes that structures and leadership be sufficiently adaptive, indeed *transformational*: so that, to quote a participant, a "9-to-5 organization may turn instantly into a 24-7 format" when it finds itself under stress. More fundamentally, it requires a culture of *genuine empowerment*, including in its legal and career ramifications, across the organization.

The resiliency of narratives

Organizational flexibility, adaptive hierarchies, and individual fortitude will be of little help, however, if collective dynamics in unconventional crises find themselves poisoned by the blurring of foundational narratives: in other words, if a company's employees, or other critical members of its human environment, struggle to retain a clear understanding of *what it is they are fighting for* in the first place, and what the endgame will look like—at what point they can expect relief, and from whom.

Unconventional crisis cells such as the RRF provide precious input in this respect. They will keep their sights squarely on the "big picture," i.e. provide an overview of response structures within the organization, and the state of the "rest of the world" outside of it: thereby ensuring that the organization's collective awareness goes beyond the blinding effect of "red lights" going off throughout the system.

The "Alignment" of International Responders

Since unconventional crises thrive in the interstices of defensive architectures, in ill-designed interfaces among their constituent parts, international systems provide an even broader target than do their domestic counterparts.

While lethal risks, within individual countries, lie in the blind spots of existing, static hierarchies, concepts, legislation, and cross-sector relations, the international scene for the main part is an anarchical mosaic of stakeholders, where the problem is not that leadership structures, prevalent doctrines and norms are *inadequate* to the situation, but rather that they are *lacking* altogether. Even the few tentative principles that have structured the field of international response, such as the tacit but seemingly self-evident difference between "aid exporters" and "aid importers," have been proven to be self-defeating by events like Katrina. In this Hobbesian world, barely tempered by valuable, yet most often merely inchoate efforts towards global governance, the mantra of coordination is even more unhelpful than it is in domestic contexts, as complexity of practices, motives, self-perception and vocabularies is such that though many would *coordinate*, few would be coordinat*ed*.

Faced with this quandary, a participant in our 2007 seminar had put forward the concept of *alignment* among international stakeholders as the only fitting response to anarchical and hypercomplex fields of actors. Instead of wasting precious time, resources and political capital in futile efforts to identify "natural" leaders of international response efforts, and to ensure that "coordinatees" close ranks around them, the argument suggests that the priority should go to establishing a basic, common purpose, operational norms, and terminological clarity—thereby creating a strategic *"magnetic field"* that will prod responders to define their own objectives and remit in mutually compatible ways, *without ever* needing explicitly to "compare notes" with one another, let alone falling under anyone else's command.

One year on, a colleague summarized his view of the "problem with international coordination" when he explained that

> "Coordination has been a controversial word. There will never be full agreement on its actual meaning. Though all want to see some form of leadership emerge, some—especially large organizations, whether the UN, NGOs, or others—definitely do *not* want to be coordinated or led. The stakeholders simply are too numerous, and diverse—increasingly so: at global, regional, national, and local levels. And there hasn't been much if any coordination or even communication among those actors: leading to duplication of efforts, gaps (as there certainly have been areas where *nobody* wanted to do anything) and competition for resources."

Coordination mechanisms

The EU platform

In the field of crisis management and civil protection as on other issues, the EU offers useful, though unavoidably flawed examples of structural efforts aiming to pull off the tight-rope exercise of coordinating twenty-seven member states while respecting their sovereignty. Most notably, the Community's Civil Protection Mechanism, and its Monitoring and Information Center, were established in 2001 to create a single radar screen, combining data provided by member states' early warning systems; while also coordinating and disseminating information on needs assessment, available assets, and ongoing response efforts in the wake of disasters, in order to eschew, or at least reduce duplication, gaps, and inopportune initiatives.

The UN platform

Similarly, within the UN framework, the lineaments of a structure have been put in place such as would clarify remits and reduce interstices or duplication in response efforts. Under the leadership of former Coordinator for Humanitarian Affairs Jan Egeland, a Humanitarian Response Review in 2004 introduced a number of structural reforms that aimed to ensure a more coordinated, fluid response system across the UN and among NGOs. Most notable was the creation of functional "clusters" (such as emergency shelters, water and sanitation, education, telecommunication, logistics, etc.), each falling under the notional lead of a specific UN agency or other NGO; while the Office of the Coordinator for Humanitarian Affairs (OCHA) became the overall hub into which the cluster "spokes" connect. Meanwhile, the allocation of financial resources and the definition of remits also were rationalized through the introduction of "Consolidated Appeals Processes" (CAPs), and the establishment of a Central Emergency Response Fund (CERF). On the ground, the UN system strives to ensure coordination among responders through "humanitarian coordinators" who head inclusive "Country Teams"—or attempt to do so.

In addition, a flurry of initiatives also has endeavored to provide a basic institutional, normative and legal framework for inter-NGO coordination, be they the InterAgency Standing Committee, NGO consortia such as InterAction, the International Council of Voluntary Agencies, the Global Humanitarian Platform, the Good Humanitarian Donorship Initiative, etc.

The value of those tools by and large is indisputable: as always in the case of UN mechanisms, arguments that would draw a blanket indictment from occasional failings and frustrating limitations are facile and short-sighted. However, even within the framework of the UN—the most likely to provide best practices in global governance and international coordination—these concepts and tools have proven eminently controversial, and have elicited considerable push-back: as "Consolidated Appeals" in particular have fallen prey to political gamesmanship within certain recipient countries, and have not always prevented the deleterious effects of inter-agency turf wars and competition over funding. Frequent NGO reluctance to accept the "straightjacket" inherent in some of these tools, which threaten to deprive them of their prized (indeed sometimes mandated) independence, illustrates the difficulty of attempting to *coordinate* international actors through structural or regulatory means. In addition, it remains doubtful whether these UN or global humanitarian initiatives can come to include a broader spectrum of international actors in the face of unconventional crises.

For instance, a participant noted that the concept of "clusters" tends to create a problematic chasm among NGOs' and states' structures and glossaries, such as threatens to compromise their capacity to interact, or indeed "*align*":

> "Clusters have been developed out of humanitarian institutions that do not match states' setup. We have to look very carefully at the lack of overlap between global NGOs' analysis, and state structures. For example, we have a global cluster on *shelter*: well, there aren't usually 'Ministries of shelter'! The clusters have broken down 'health' into a nutrition cluster, a water cluster, and a health cluster. But medical professionals know that public health requires an integrated approach. And so, you're seeing a tension between the organizational principles of states, and those of the global humanitarian community. And if we're talking about ensuring *alignment*, I think we're going down a road that will lead to more, rather than fewer disconnects."

Indeed, this and other concepts were often developed *de facto* to exclude national or local authorities which NGOs mistrusted out of a poor analytical distinction among competent, failing, and failed states.

> "The CERF, for instance, is restricted to UN agencies. And so you're putting more and more money towards these global institutions that are not necessarily running their operations in close consultation with local authorities. Our mantra as NGOs is that we 'support local authorities': and yet our institutions increasingly have taken over roles of leadership, potentially undermining local capacities. So I would argue that if we want to talk about *alignment*, we really need to think very carefully about how we organize our respective sets of mechanisms, and how they're going to intersect with what already exists."

In the same way, recent UN reforms have done little to ensure more consistent and effective interaction between humanitarian efforts and the private sector—even though the latter, as a participant insisted, often finds itself on the front line of immediate response efforts in the period between the occurrence of an unconventional crisis and the first arrival of NGO or state assets on the scene. Thus, following Katrina, private companies were forced to bridge this chronological and operational gap with no clear sense of the nature of NGO strategies. "Global humanitarian agencies have probably made the mistake of seeing the private sector solely as a contributor of financial support—as opposed to a key partner that controls so much of critical infrastructure."

Indeed, humanitarian organizations have embedded cultural or conceptual chasms among sectors by developing sets of standards which cannot easily be reconciled with incentive structures or the *modus operandi* of other stakeholders. "For humanitarian agencies, there is a problem in interacting with new players: namely how to make sure that they agree with and stand by humanitarian standards like the Sphere Project, Humanitarian Accountability Partnership International, and others."

From unity of command to unity of effort

These examples of exclusive coordination mechanisms hint at a broader issue, namely the fact that structural attempts to broaden coordination platforms or indeed create "global parliaments" *must* fail in the face of the complexity that characterizes unconventional crises and the international field of relevant stakeholders. "It is virtually impossible: no coordination mechanism can remain effective when you have that many actors." New information technologies only push back, but do not altogether transcend, the inherent limitations of such structural initiatives: "virtual platforms" can be broader than their physical counterparts, but must eventually discriminate between insiders and outsiders, lest they implode under the pressures brought about by their own complexity.

> "During the Tsunami, thirty-five countries showed up, one after the other, and every time somebody showed up we had to go back to the beginning again, and get everybody on board. And some of us had a lot more experience on these issues than others, but we had to get everyone's green light—and people were in the room who weren't authorized to make decisions for their government, so they would have

to send messages back to their capitals, and they would get the answer back three days later."

As a participant noted, any decision-making process that trusts coordination rather than "alignment" to face hypercomplex challenges requires that stakeholders' egos "be left outside the door." While he successfully flagged the problem, he did not draw the unmistakable conclusion—that this surely entails the ultimate demise of all over-ambitious attempts to coordinate international stakeholders, as egos in fact *will not* be kept in check. Similarly, the ideal-typical coordination mechanism that he described seems inherently unattainable:

> "You've got to put the right people in the room, and then somebody has to chair it, and to do it in an effective and strong manner, and then everybody's got to agree like a Cabinet: 'that's fine, we had our vote, we'll follow the major-ity view and get going on this.' To me, that is the essence of the problem."

It certainly is the essence of the problem: but it also suggests why the same problem, simply put, is intractable. Indeed, a top-down, structural effort to coordinate hypercomplex maps of international actors implies that

> "Incoming participants become incoming hits that impact your system. Take the case of individuals who showed up following the Tsunami or Katrina because they'd seen a TV report: how do you explain to these people that 'we have a thirty-year tradition' as to how to go about things, that 'we're the coordinators, you be the coordinatees': that's not going to work, and you'll have to make the same case over and over again."

Not only the complexity of relevant stakeholders, but also that of cultural, normative and legal frameworks, dooms coordination efforts past a certain threshold. Thus, "there is a contradiction inherent in CERF: as the donors want to see speed in disbursements and initiatives, while at the same time, the same governments clamor for 'accountabil-ity, standards, and due process.'"

What is needed is to turn emerging unconventional participants from *incoming hits* into *building blocks*, by abandoning the illusion that increased structural coordination by itself can be the answer, and striving instead to create intangible *alignment* among stakeholders. In other words, we must move from a culture of *unity of command* towards one that prioritizes *unity of effort*.

Structure and culture of mutual aid

Transnational mutual aid agreements provide a useful example of a mechanism whose value, when confronting unconventional crises, has laid less in the unity of command which they had set out to create, than in the incremental emergence of a common culture that enabled unity of effort. Certainly, agreements between the Canadian and U.S. Coast Guards played a substantial role following Hurricane Katrina, as the former took over responsibilities in the U.S. Northeast to enable their American colleagues to deploy resources and manpower in areas affected by the storm. Yet, the most successful, though unheralded cross-border initiatives came from Canadian and American officials "breaking the rules" to develop *ad hoc* solutions based on tacit mutual understanding and a subjacent common culture.

> "Canada sent an urban Search and Rescue Team in the South, and they just sort of packed their bags and left: they had a local contact. And the Canadian military just jumped the gun and came down, and told the government afterwards what they were doing. The Louisiana State governor signed a waiver to create more accreditations in Louisiana for Canadian doctors who arrived on the scene and couldn't treat patients otherwise. The truth is, we improvised our assistance to the United States. There was no systemic approach."

Alignment

Core culture and coalescence

Though the concept of alignment can often seem frustratingly intangible, even impressionistic, the example of joint Canada-U.S. crisis response culture demonstrates that it is in fact built upon very pragmatic foundations: namely considerable discipline, preparation, and trust among (at least) a kernel of stakeholders, proportional to the chaotic nature of the environment in which they operate.

Such core responders will contribute to the process of alignment by creating a stable focal point around which others can coalesce, or which they, at least, can utilize as a rare bearing to determine their own strategy and behavior. Core stakeholders will also provide others with pragmatic best practices that do not presume to dictate or even interpret anyone's motives, nor to impose a specific operational template, and therefore hold no hierarchical implications.

Alignment, then, can only succeed if such groups of core responders develop a culture that combines disciplined training drills with operational and analytical flexibility, rather than opposing them. Again, the solution lies in stakeholders seeing intellectual curiosity and out-of-the-box initiatives not as threats, but as assets; not as *moments*, but as *processes*.

A participant noted that "humanitarian organizations have developed a common vocabulary, because a lot of them respond over and over again to the same crises, so that there is a built-up level of trust and mutual understanding." Similarly, a colleague hailed UN-led efforts to set up cross-silo platforms and training drills, such as the short-lived "Business Roundtable". Certainly, on the international scene, the challenge inherent in such drills is only compounded, as there is a fine line between utilizing them to nurture adaptive responses to the unconventional, such as can contribute to the alignment of complex maps of responders, and drawing static bodies of knowledge from these exercises in order to close ranks around the "illusion of certainty" to the exclusion of all unconventional actors. Yet in the end, only discipline, and the cultivation of a flexible, adaptive, inquisitive comfort zone among colleagues, can draw alignment out of conceptual impressionism and turn it into a tangible organizational force; as it will create core groups and endow them with the critical mass necessary to exert a gravitational pull on other, independent stakeholders, through interpersonal relationships, instincts, common terminology and standards.

In other words, there is no zero-sum game between "coordination" and "alignment," no inherent contradiction in terms between the two concepts: only a deadly illusion in the proposition that the former suffices to meet the challenge of unconventional crises any more than does intangible "alignment" deprived of all underlying structure.

Incentive structures: leverage and narrative

In concrete terms, "gravitational pull" can take many forms simultaneously. More intangible factors such as the prestige and experience of core groups will combine with pragmatic considerations such as their operational capacity, monopoly on rare assets, or control over logistical "bottlenecks" in response efforts; indeed the very *success* of these core groups will be their most powerful contribution towards aligning other responders along a "magnetic field" that they will have created. Yet an additional factor lies in the development of *incentive structures* that will permeate the response environment, and increase the odds that unrelated stakeholders will adopt mutually compatible and broadly complementary approaches.

One of our participants lauded business models as useful templates to develop intelligent incentive structures—the paragon of *"non-hierarchical"* coordination mechanisms, diametrically opposed to military approaches: "in the business world, there's no statutory mandate, there are no ranks on people's shoulders; they will do something because there's some benefit to doing it."

As he put it, unconventional crises create response environments "with all kinds of different 'currencies' that stimulate stakeholders. And it doesn't have to be money. It can be skillful allocation of visible 'primacy' to flatter responders' egos. Another one is information: you can provide information to NGOs in 'payment' for collaboration, cooperation." Indeed, such "payments" or incentives can take many other forms, reflecting the variety of rare assets and operational bottlenecks that we mentioned above.

This view, however, still proceeds from the premise that *someone*—seemingly, for our participant, the public sector—will be the "natural leader" of complex international response efforts, and therefore will find itself in an uncontested and monopolistic position to "dish out" precious "currency" as it pleases in order to organize a coherent, Cartesian incentive architecture. Such a structure can easily devolve from incentivization into tacit coercion, or a "carrots-and-sticks" system. More to the point, it does not resolve the challenge at hand, namely the fact that unconventional crises will create chaotic response environments in which no single stakeholder can define incentive frameworks on its own, or control enough "critical currency" to sustain them—as prevailing anarchy (sometimes indeed rivalry) among responders will undermine all efforts to exert predictable leverage through such means.

What is needed, then, is to turn from the "currencies of incentivization" to its *narrative underpinnings*: to enable the emergence of an interpretation of the crisis that will be broad enough to be shared by all, transversal enough to avoid cultural bents or subjacent hierarchical implications; and will simply specify the *identity of the victims*, the *role of responders*, and the nature of *success* in a way that will allow unconnected stakeholders to infer their *own incentive structures*, their own carrots and sticks, from this basic set of paradigms.

Again, unconventional events will make it impossible for one single responder to impose such an overarching interpretation, as others simply will not *listen*. Participants suggested two solutions to this quandary: first, sharing intelligence across silos and governance strata; second, reinstating victims at the center of the narrative of their own disaster.

Pervasive information

The first way to avoid an unhelpful competition among potential narratives is to ensure that information about the crisis at hand is shared among all stakeholders, so that all can come to a broadly compatible—if not similar—understanding of the challenge, based on the most fundamental commonality among responders: their appreciation of the thin red line between victims' death and survival. Certainly this will not circumvent all spoilers: but it will at least thin their ranks, and shed a crude light on their real motives.

Thus the UN has developed mechanisms that can usefully contribute to the alignment of responders, in the form of intelligent and adaptive cross-silo information systems. In addition to information centralized by e.g. OCHA, UNDP, UNHCR, and WFP, the UN's "Who Does What Where" databases set up a basic mapping of complex fields of actors, and thereby provide the lineaments of the "magnetic field" that we describe, such as can reduce overlap and increase compatibility among remits and allocations of assets. It is illuminating, indeed, that this "non-structural" mechanism, which entirely eschews the loaded questions involved in discriminating among "leaders" and "followers," has proven much less controversial than UN coordination systems listed above, such as CAPs or the CERF. The same effort towards "information alignment" is evident in another database, ReliefWeb, which, though administered by OCHA, does not impose UN pre-eminence upon its variegated users. Country-specific Humanitarian Information Centers also have been created to provide single point of contact, web-based sources of cross-silo information.

UN-led efforts are laudable, but insufficient. They are limited in scope, and reflect a specific operational culture whose premises are not universally applicable. In addition, the information they provide in effect has mostly been utilized, and sometimes can only be accessed by humanitarian professionals from countries that traditionally have been "exporters of aid." Such databases, then, reach their limits in circumstances such as Katrina, when traditional paradigms of global aid agencies, and the comfort of working among trusted partners, are instantly overwhelmed. For all the outpouring of goodwill—or in part because of it—the international response to the storm, as we noted above, was characterized by pervasive duplication, gaps in cross-silo awareness, and posturing among stakeholders whose inopportune offers of help became part of the problem rather than of the solution.

When confronting the chaotic, hypercomplex environments left in the wake of unconventional disruptions, logistical databases can only meet the challenge if they enable the bottom-up coalescence of anarchical fields of users that social networking sites provide in other contexts. Our seminar, then, undertook a concerted effort to examine what such a database should look like, and who could in fact host it. The answer to both questions reflects the proposition that this instrument should eschew static, bureaucratic, centralized, and exclusive templates. Simply put, it can only take the shape of a portal synthesizing information provided by others, and enabling intelligent access to their respective systems. No single organization, not even the UN (or specifically its Disaster Assessment and Coordination team), can credibly be tasked with the oversight and logistical management of the mechanism. The tool should rather be inspired by the paradigms that underlie "Web 2.0," striving to shape anarchical fields of stakeholders into fluid, yet eminently actionable dynamics: a "Craigslist, a clearing-house, a matchmaker, a node of humanitarian aid."

In addition to operational assets such as tents, blankets, medicine etc., the ideal "portal" should also provide concerted information on more tactical and strategic resources, such as rosters of available, competent personnel, and shipping or—crucially—airlift assets; while also enabling a dialogue among complex fields of stakeholders about the *nature of the crisis* itself, thus creating the most potent guarantee against groupthink and inaccurate labels.

Enhancing local capacity: bottom-up alignment

Pervasive, "anarchical" information-sharing among incoming responders, however, still fails to acknowledge or utilize the mechanism that could most effectively ensure their alignment: namely the emergence of a common narrative from the bottom-up—as *victims themselves* would define who they are, what they need, what the objectives of response ought to be, and the nature of success; thus establishing an unassailable narrative that would *trickle up* among all outside responders. In other words, victims themselves would make up a "core group" whose culture would orient global response efforts, and around which other stakeholders would coalesce.

This entails that local communities should be granted joint ownership of their own crisis, and of their own needs assessment, resulting in a demand-based, rather than supply-based dynamics.

> "Moving away from terminologies that describe them as 'victims' or 'beneficiaries,' or even—oddly—as 'outsiders' to response efforts, how can we make sure that those people, through better preparedness, through capacity building, are able to articulate response efforts themselves, to *help organize* international responders. How can they be at the center of the disaster; how can they have the ability, as

they have the *right*, to control the 'outsiders' who are coming into *their* disaster? And for them to be, if not in the driving seat, at least very much involved in decision-making processes. So it goes much beyond the mantra of '72-hour self-sufficiency.'"

Enabling *bottom-up alignment* by restoring victims to the center of incentive structures and interpretation of crisis is not only, then, a moral imperative, but also, on a strategic plane, the most convincing route to meet the challenge of hypercomplexity in international response efforts. Practical implications to bring about this change are certainly daunting—though it seems in part unattainable because of cultural reluctance on the part of upper-tier decision-makers to contemplate the objective.

In practical terms, though, the first step towards enhancing local control over response efforts is clear: it lies with stronger local input into international assessment and early warning mechanisms; as those bridge the gap between affected countries and the international community of responders, and therefore foreshadow and shape the cultural paradigms that will dominate response efforts. Victims, then, can only acquire ownership of their own disasters if early warning structures grant them ownership of their own risk assessment.

Education, Training, and the Culture of Leaders

The problem with leadership culture

In our section on the "certainty of the unthinkable," we highlighted the differences, and interdependence, between two factors that account for leaders' frequent inability to anticipate unconventional crises, and to react effectively when they occur: individual psychology and organizational pressures.

Some of our participants saw a zero-sum game in this dichotomy: claiming that structural pressures and failings fully account for any apparent individual irresolution in the face of the "unthinkable"; that leaders, in the end, have nothing to learn in order to improve their performance:

> "Very often warning signals will go off, and *nothing happens*. And the question comes down to: why is that the case? And the most frequent answer would be: 'it's leadership.' But I would argue that the issue is *not* leadership: it is not the fact that senior officials within our respective agencies do not understand the nature of the decisions they're being asked to make. It is that there are strong incentives for them *not* to act. And these incentives come from our political process. We have citizens who seem to be much more interested and willing to reward people who respond *ex post*, than they do in rewarding people who actually prevented problems in a proactive way. And it seems to me that we can jump up and down and say: 'we would like our leaders to show more courage and flexibility' when confronting unconventional crises. But until we change those incentives, that's not going to happen."

A colleague seconded the thought, noting that difficulties in "turning early warning into early action" were "a political and financial problem: because spending political capital and obtaining funding for preparedness, even if you know an event is coming up, is not as attractive as getting involved after a tsunami, a flood, or an earthquake."

According to this view, instead of focusing on leaders, training efforts aiming to effect a cultural shift should therefore be directed at the greater public itself—at least in democratic polities where the public determines political incentive structures.

> "We need to focus on citizens, so that we get society to *demand* from their political leaders that they act before crisis hits. If we can educate people to *expect* a better outcome, then maybe we can change the way in which decisions are made in the polling booths, and get the incentives that will drive leaders to act more proactively. And I would argue that, while this is particularly germane for the public sector, to the extent that private sector actors have to respond to investors, they may be facing some of the same problems."

Certainly, taking into account organizational and collective dimensions helpfully drives the analysis beyond an exclusive and facile focalization on individual failings. However, organizational drivers should not blind us either to the very real problems that lie with inadequate individual responses to unconventional events among leaders themselves. It is simply not good enough to give them an easy "pass" by arguing, as a participant did, that "slowly, their awareness of unconventional challenges has improved... and we need to recognize that it is very challenging for them to adapt... but in the past ten years, I have seen slow progress."

Why the bar should be set so low, why "slow progress"—itself questionable—should seem satisfactory, was not explained; the proposition indeed can seem shocking when other professionals with critical responsibilities—military personnel come to mind—are held to much more stringent standards as to their capacity to meet all challenges, irrespective of their cultural "discomfort" in doing so. Most participants, then, vigorously objected to a rosy appreciation of leaders' investment in unconventional challenges, highlighting repeated instances in which upper-tier executives had simply skipped ambitious training sessions, and thereby had given unmistakable signs that such events were nowhere near the top of their agenda. Even the proposition that "political leaders don't go out of their way to find other perspectives, but often welcome them when they are brought in" was seen to be too generous.

Highlighting individual inadequacies certainly does not entail that analysis must devolve into finger-pointing, as leaders are only exemplars of the professional culture that has permeated their training. The proposition only suggests that a determined effort must be made to modify this culture: that leaders indeed have "something to learn."

The "problems with leaders' culture" were characterized in different ways by our participants. Some suggested that the challenge stemmed from the generalist outlook that is most common among elected and private sector officials, noting that "ministers have an enormous and difficult burden on their hands, as they are thrown from the generalization of politics into the particular problems of crisis"; while "business leaders typically don't have a point of reference for managing unconventional crises: they're focused on business, full stop." Others approached the problem from a different—though not incompatible—standpoint, underlining the complex ramifications of crisis, as it is "difficult for leaders to tackle all the dimensions of unconventional crises, from public health, to political, economic, social, and diplomatic implications. The task truly is superhuman, and can only be addressed through teamwork: but leaders find this challenging."

A consensus, however, emerged among colleagues to push the argument further, and put in question the structure, the value system itself, that underpins leaders' culture, and indeed their selection and promotion: thereby implying that the challenge is one of "changing leaders' mindset" altogether—their "mental framework, culture, creativity, emotional response, and leadership skills."

Commenting on the 2008 food crisis, and the resulting riots that affected several countries at the time, a participant highlighted baffling contradictions in leaders' intellectual skills, and hinted at cultural obstacles:

> "This is not rocket science; anyone could have seen it coming, and so many specialists had actually examined many of the pieces that are leading to where we are right now. And yet, it still caught us flat-footed. For all our thoughtfulness,

and all the money that we spend in analysis, in collecting data, in communicating on the risks: we still seem unable to connect the dots, and get ahead of the curve. We have so much information, so much intelligence around the table, and yet such a hard time tackling unconventional crises: and it *is* about a failure of leadership, and it *is* a failure of imagination, and they continue to plague us."

At bottom lies a simple question: namely why,

"Though 'entrepreneurial thinkers' now have identified the challenges of unconventional crises, we still are lacking 'venture capitalists' within governments and other institutions who can acknowledge the issue, and are willing to risk the capital—whether political, financial, organizational—to tackle it."

Or, as another colleague put it,

"Why we can't seem to take unconventional threats seriously; why the most common response among leaders remains sheer denial; why they and the public alike still are surprised when these risks materialize; why, in the wake of disasters, we take refuge in a fatalist outlook, or wallow in our status as 'victims of the unthinkable.' Why leaders lock themselves into silo-specific dynamics, and a 'planning arms race.' Why we aren't nimble enough to create ad-hoc 'alchemies' among organizations."

The same participant answered his own question by setting his sight squarely on cultural failings at the individual level, which structural pressures partly explain, but do not *explain away*:

"I am looking at those who in principle should be *leaders*; and what I see, by and large, are mere *managers*. And they are brilliant, they are highly educated: the problem does not stem from lack of intellectual capacity—but lack of conviction, lack of imagination. Today we are dealing with leaders who, most often, no longer know how to clarify situations; who cannot identify the crux of an issue; who cannot define *priorities*—they always deal with *emergencies*, but have lost the ability to establish *priorities*. And they struggle to produce courageous decision-making, audacious initiatives. In the final analysis, then, there is a real problem with the education of our leaders."

A colleague saw leaders who are "disengaged from crisis management, and who are far from convinced of the need to improve their organization's performance in this respect." A participant reflected on "leaders' paralysis in the face of unconventional threats, which isn't always explained by their insidious nature: when you look at risks involved in asbestos, in smoking, the problem was visible twenty or thirty years before political leaders acted on it"; while another described "executives who make knee-jerk decisions, because the intensity, the volatility, the chaotic nature of unconventional events destabilizes everyone," as "leaders go through the shocking realization that there's been very little preparation for the actual event they're facing, that it's too late to dream up assets that do not exist, and that they are going to have to make do with *exactly* what they have."

Paralysis, destabilization and *shock* are indeed crucial words. A participant talks of the "stun effect" or shellshock that he has observed time and again among leaders and organizations that had refused to prepare for the unconventional, out of a culturally ingrained reluctance even to envisage it.

"It seems to me that the crucial issue in preparing leaders is precisely that unconventional crises trigger enormous discomfort among those in charge of response. As soon as crisis erupts, collective intelligence somehow finds itself paralyzed; and communication becomes impossible, while leadership vanishes. Officials grab for dear life onto basic tools that they were taught would work. This reflects the prevalent tendency in the training of leaders: as their teachers adopt a magisterial posture, claiming to hold, and divulge, all the right answers, the right tools, 'what you are going to do.' And then leaders go home with a thick file of 'best practices,' and they think 'it's all in there': but it doesn't work!—because these ready-made tools will be circumvented and made irrelevant by crisis.

Instead, the priority should be to prepare leaders to confront the unknown, tackle complexity: and *not* to be paralyzed or stunned by it. And if we don't do this, if we stick to conventional academic teaching, or conventional training practices, then as soon as you're hit by a Katrina, the reaction among leaders is: 'I don't have a roadmap to do anything about this; let's wait until it conforms to *my* niche.' We have to develop a different form of training: train people for the unknown, and *not* for what we know."

Again, the point in framing the issue at the level of individual cultural inadequacies is not to ascribe blame, but to find practical mechanisms that will resolve the problem. Indeed, as a participant argued, "We have to stop opposing 'experts' and 'leaders'; on the contrary, they must collaborate so the former can provide the latter with methods and concepts that will improve decision-making processes."

Considerable experience in the field has led our participants to propose, develop, and test pragmatic training and educational formats that reflect their appreciation of the problem, and give flesh to the argument. Though highlighting the importance of cultural reform in improving leadership performance in unconventional events may seem overly intangible or even impractical, the "new training methods" advocated by our participants can be described in some detail.

Unconventional training

The key to avoiding stun effects in the face of the "unthinkable" lies, conventionally enough, in recreating a comfort zone; not, however, by nurturing the "comfort of certainty": but rather the capacity of leaders to thrive in a chaotic universe, among unresolved questions, and under time pressure.

The United Kingdom in particular provides examples of training mechanisms aiming to

"develop disciplined processes that enable pragmatic decision-making, and allow rapid learning and innovation; while also ensuring that leaders have the time, and cultivate the will, to work outside the box. The key words are breadth of thinking; the willingness to learn and innovate; appetite for risk; being prepared to confront the inevitable; and having a very good supporting process that allows decisions to be made at a pace that meets the speed of the disruption."

The foot-and-mouth crisis highlighted the difference in performance that stems from agencies' unequal capacity to produce rhythmic decision-making in hypercomplex environments, reflecting their respective training and culture.

"The U.K. put a military brigade headquarters into the Agriculture Department; because they just *did not know* how to run a complex decision-making process, whereas the military know how to deal with that enormous wave of unexpected information, how to organize it. Which doesn't mean that the military took the lead; they merely delivered a supporting process. Politicians, epidemiologists, veterinarians remained in command, but what they didn't have was experience of handling that enormous influx of undifferentiated information. They just *froze*; while the military simply didn't freeze."

However, relying on partnerships with outside organizations that happen to have nurtured adequate behavioral patterns is at best a stopgap solution. Salvation must come from all leaders being incrementally sensitized to the implications of chaotic environments, and their proper role within them, so they can themselves eschew unconventional stun effects. For instance,

"Putting leaders in the middle of the machinery of response, and letting them experience just what it's like. Making them sit there, and go through the decision-making that will take hijacked airliners out of the sky before they hit a capital city. We can't train them to understand the technical capabilities involved: they have to trust the trained emergency managers. But they will get to know the people, the likely parameters of the system. They will learn that there is great merit in thinking beyond the envelope that is normally theirs; in understanding the broader picture, the dependencies of their particular organization, the role that it plays within networks, the traffic that it carries, supply, demand, resources that it absolutely needs."

Such training formats therefore have unique value in helping leaders—most notably elected officials—"understand what their *role* is within response efforts—and where the *limits* are to their role. Because response systems repeatedly have been broken asunder by officials going beyond their proper remit out of political motivations; and once you break that response system, it takes weeks to reconstruct it." Or, as another participant noted,

> "In the beginning of Katrina, one of the biggest obstacles to providing service was that leaders did not operate at the levels that were appropriate for them. They were all over the place. Senior leadership was down at the operational level, which was disruptive and confusing. The President of the United States came into the operation room of my organization—and stopped operations for half a day."

At bottom, the challenge is a simple matter of helping leaders to keep their eyes wide open when contemplating the "unthinkable": and doing so by having them understand that it need not be the "abyss," it need not spell disaster, if only they seek their salvation in mastering disciplined movement, rather than in digging trenches that will be their graves.

This entails that training exercises eschew the pursuit of symbolic reassurance of the *status quo*; or competition among participants' egos, as all seek to reassert their status by suggesting that nothing can truly be "unconventional" to them. The temptation can be circumvented by grouping participants into unconventional teams, thus transcending individual posturing; by making it clear that "an exercise which runs smoothly cannot be useful"; and by laying out scenarios that "push the envelope" and "deliberately throw things at people" to highlight the most challenging impacts of unconventional crises; while preventing denial or evasion by setting the ground rule that these scenarios *cannot be questioned*.

Some organizations have tentatively been moving towards "high impact" planning: FEMA, for instance, has developed a Catastrophe Planning Initiative that looks at "previously unimaginable scenarios" such as reiterations of a New Madrid earthquake, "Long Island express," or catastrophic failure of the North Eastern power grid; an eruption of Mount Rainier; and persistent flooding in Florida following a breach of the Herbert Hoover dike. But these efforts remain marginal—and may in fact be counter-productive if they merely draw up static plans against such contingencies, and attempt to "tame" unconventional events rather than leaders' destabilization when confronting them. In any case, most organizations, in all sectors, "still are averse to opening themselves up to those scenarios."

We highlighted the "problem with plans" in our 2008 report, drawing a distinction between behavioral planning, which unhelpfully purports to dictate each responder's steps when facing disaster, though chaotic environments will break apart this neat "chain of actions"—and *resource-based* planning, which sets out to identify fundamental building blocks from which stakeholders and victims themselves can reconstruct a rational response. The argument need not be repeated here: a participant made a similar point when he noted that his organization

> "was moving away from scenario building: as no scenario ever works out in the way you think it will; and there are just too many complex contingencies. So there's been a paradigm shift here. We now map out hazards and risks, analyze them, analyze our operational processes, assess how critical our functions are, how long of a downtime each one can sustain."

Denial in front of the unconventional will further be eschewed if organizations nurture a process that looks back at actual crises and the challenges they raised—not however through blue-ribbon commissions of enquiry whose reports will simply collect dust, and whose "lessons learned" will go unheeded, but by setting up cross-silo, bottom-up "crisis parliaments" that will collect the views of leaders, employees, and partners alike. Thus a private company, following Katrina, held what it called a "hurricane summit" that included all of the field personnel involved in the response, comprising individuals who had made crucial decisions through the crisis irrespective of their hierarchical position.

The point is well taken that the preceding paragraphs only describe an agenda to modify leaders' culture, yet not *per se* a solution to tenacious mental blocks, or to spoilers' refusal to even envisage reform. As a participant noted, "the effectiveness of training entirely depends on whether you're dealing with people who go along for the ride. If you're looking at government or private sector officials who remain cynical and unconvinced, training will not change a thing."

At the individual level, mental blocks can have various causes: whether uneasiness to look beyond one's comfort zone; or the fear to expose one's limits in the face of the unconventional. Another problematic factor can be the belief—widespread among elected politicians—that the same resourcefulness, instinct, and improvisation that underpinned their political career will be more effective than tedious training sessions to guarantee their effectiveness if the "unthinkable" occurs—while also being more likely to turn them into heroic figures, and endow them with the resulting political capital, if they should indeed be successful or appear to be.

Three paths can be followed to circumvent these obstacles. First, leaders' concern that preparing for unconventional contingencies will unavoidably shed unflattering light on their skills can be alleviated by maintaining a tight secret on their performance in training drills, and smoothing out scenarios and options just enough so that leaders never utterly fail in exercises. Second, their reluctance can be ascribed to a permeating, antiquated leadership culture which individuals simply cannot transcend: in which case we must turn our sights to the next generation of upcoming leaders. Lastly, the case can be made, as indeed it was made above, that leaders' mental blocks in front of unconventional training reflect organizational pressures that feed into this reluctance.

These pressures can result from the fact that an organization imposes upon leaders priorities and mental frameworks that discourage their "divestment" into preparations for abnormal contingencies—indeed even prevent them from *perceiving* the problem altogether, as it doesn't relate to their remit, their radar screen, or their vocabulary. As a participant explained,

"Leaders will only be convinced that anticipating unconventional and catastrophic events not only ranks among their responsibilities, but *ranks first*, if the challenge can be explained in terms that will resonate with them, whether industrial or managerial: namely, if we can highlight the added value, the competitive edge, that preparing for these events can hold for their organization."

As we noted above, however, organizational pressures can also stem from unhelpful expectations among leaders' subordinates and the greater public alike, which create a cultural and political environment in which preparing for the unconventional seems like a waste of leaders' time, or a threat to their status. Efforts to modify culture and training practices, then, must take on a collective *as well as* individual dimension. A participant noted that leaders in his country were apparently more prepared than others to take a proactive part in training exercises as "they know that the day after the event, they're going to be facing political scrutiny about their level of readiness; they're actually going to be in front of their political opponents; and that focuses a few minds." What "focuses leaders' minds" on unconventional threats, then, ultimately is the greater public's expectation that preparing for them is a quintessential part of leaders' remit and responsibility—*as it also is the responsibility of the public itself.*

Unconventional drills and exercises therefore must be the tip of the iceberg, the momentary manifestation of continuous training that will be nurtured throughout organizations among and across silos. Not only the culture of leaders, but that of their subordinates, must be challenged to effect a change in organizational expectations and incentives structures that weigh upon decision-makers when confronting unconventional disruptions. A fundamental aspect of this change must come from permeating awareness of an organization's interdependence with others, for instance through the creation of career incentives for mid-level employees to spend time working for partners of their home organization. However, as a participant deplored, "though there is a push at the senior level to encourage interagency understanding, to work with one another, communicate, do rotations: at the *lowest* level of government, there still is a tendency to indoctrinate incoming employees in their own department's views."

Unconventional leadership skills

This subjacent, organization-wide, cross-silo culture cannot be the result of occasional drills, but only of generational efforts to educate crisis managers at all levels in specialized schools. FEMA's Emergency Management Institute has become the paragon of institutional efforts to set up cross-silo educational programs that strive to develop unconventional thinking, together with more traditional crisis management skills, among students recruited from a wide spectrum of backgrounds: aiming to create a specific culture and know-how that can trickle up, down, and outward through other levels of government and private sector. Indeed,

> "Emergency managers are in a position to influence politicians and policy-makers above them who rotate on a more frequent basis: they can inculcate leadership in decision-makers, with an ethics based on the realization of the need to prepare for hypercomplex events. FEMA is training people who can work both upstream and downstream, and who go on to have careers not only in government, but in private corporations as well. Therefore, they can bring new cultural frameworks and experience-based information into a great variety of organizations; and can help dispel or mitigate the reluctance of top-level decision-makers to confront unconventional threats."

"Trickle-up" cultural changes were highlighted by a participant who argued that "if you consistently expose a broader and broader group, at ever higher levels, to unconventional challenges, the willingness for top leadership to invest themselves in the process increases, because you broaden their area of comfort as you develop the organization's exposure to these issues over a number of years."

Changes in mid-level culture and know-how, therefore, are certainly a useful complement, even in some respect a prerequisite, for similar cultural and behavioral shifts among upper-tier leaders—especially as unconventional crises will prod the emergence of effective leadership from unexpected sources. But changes restricted to this intermediate stratum are not *per se* sufficient, if only because the persistence of mental blocks among top leadership can undermine constructive cultural evolutions at all lower levels of an organization.

The stakes of unconventional risks today are such that upper leadership exerts unique, irreplaceable leverage on organizations' response, for good or evil. "Not all layers can take critical decisions when faced, for instance, with the recent financial crisis and the prospect of instantly losing billions of dollars: this remains the exclusive remit of a minute group of top leaders." Only they can restore confidence, a sense of collective purpose, a framework for understanding chaotic environments; as only they can trigger cross-strata panic if they show themselves entirely unprepared to respond. In other words, "training mid-level emergency managers is not good enough: we need decision-makers themselves to acknowledge that they must prepare for the unconventional." The two processes, indeed, should be symbiotic—which is at best a remote prospect today, when, as a participant noted, "there is a real disconnect between political leadership and mid-level, permanent staff, which only becomes exacerbated in crisis situations when you have to make decisions based on relationships that have been cultivated on a daily basis, but barely exist across organizational layers."

In any case, FEMA's EMI remains an isolated example, as participants agreed that no elite school of business or public affairs, whether in Europe or North America, at present trains its students to confront anything but commonplace, anticipated disruptions.

> "It is unacceptable that in terms of requirements, elite schools should set the bar so low, and suggest to their students that, once in leadership positions, they will only be confronted with routine situations—or somehow can rely upon others if something worse happens. There will be no 'firefighters' to step in and come to the rescue of upper-tier leadership. They are *it!*"

A participant, however, flagged an obstacle that still hinders efforts towards elaborating such educational programs: the lack of a synthetic "reference document" that would explicitly list the set of skills required of future leaders and crisis managers to face unconventional disruptions. Indeed, he saw the cross-silo platform convened by our seminars as a unique opportunity to draft such a consensual framework, among government, private sector, and NGO officials, but also educators and policy analysts; and called upon colleagues to build upon this promising start. Notionally, this set of skills would comprise a foundation common to all stakeholders in unconventional response, irrespective of their specific role: while *ad-hoc* subsets of competencies could be added on to reflect the spectrum of skills that runs from e.g. mid-level officials tasked with delivering technical capabilities, to leaders whose remit is broader and more strategic in nature, including the ability to run complex decision-making processes and the more intangible capacity to "marshal people's enthusiasm."

This list of skills would be eminently pragmatic, based upon real-life failings or successes. As a case in point, a participant explained that his organization took note of employees who had risen to the occasion of unconventional crises irrespective of their rank in the hierarchy: and would "bring them into the training structure, so working almost backwards: from the fact that they've proven their skills by experience, we then try to capture that, and adapt it to a technical, 'classroom' type of approach."

Tentative efforts toward the drafting and publication of such sets of unconventional skills have already begun in a U.S. context. The challenge now is "to explore these issues from a truly integrated, international point of view," and then to submit the resulting toolbox to organizations across all sectors, and to prod them to act upon it based on the credibility and prestige of the international platform of practitioners and experts that would put it forward.

In the process, however, it is imperative that this drive towards defining and summarizing "knowledge contents" *stem from* the culture shift described above, rather than becoming one more evading tactics that will find illusory comfort in the elaboration of lists and answers. Thus, a participant insisted that

> "It is certainly helpful to provide rules, beacons, capabilities, so that leaders can learn how to deal with complex information, complex logistics, etc. But this should not blind us to the real challenge, which such knowledge will

not resolve by itself: the cultural stun effect that paralyzes leaders' intelligence and decision-making when the unconventional hits."

Lists of skills will be self-defeating if this issue is not resolved first: dooming leaders either robotically to grab to this new body of knowledge—which will then have achieved nothing but replacing a set of static guidelines, a Maginot line, with another—or to tear the same document to pieces when facing the unconventional, in utter despair that it can be addressed at all.

> "*That* is the main problem. Enough with technical knowledge, with crisis communication, crisis room gadgets, enough with calling for 'more assets,' 'more plans,' 'more media training'! All this we know how to do; all this leaders are comfortable with. But what we must focus on, what still elicits reluctance, is education that will prod them to think on their feet, to deal with chaos: there is *nothing* of the sort in leaders' education at present. Nothing akin not to the professorial arrogance of military brass 'who know the answers,' but to the culture of special forces, who are taught to create intelligence in alien, confusing environments that were never *specifically* described in their training."

If the elaboration and transmission of clear sets of skills, however, takes account of the cultural challenge at hand, rather than serving to elude it, "the known and the unknown" can be mutually complementary, indeed symbiotic: as

> "Making it clear that we do have tools, based on the teachings of experience, will help leaders trust that the challenge of the unconventional can in fact be met: thus eroding their mental block. Whereas if you leave them with nothing but a daunting insight into unconventional challenges, and a call to 'be smart and adaptive' backed up by no definite toolbox, they will simply run away."

A colleague summarized the point when he argued that

"Our priority must be to 'burst the bubble of crisis': help leaders and employees to move beyond their fear of it, beyond their perception that its impact will necessarily be overwhelming. And we can only dispel the mystique of crisis through education, utilizing a basic framework of knowledge that will reassure them, help them become familiar with a toolbox which they can then transcend to recreate an intelligent, adaptive comfort zone. This is true across all strata of an organization: upper-tier managers must play their part in drills and invest themselves in this effort; but cannot succeed without equal buy-in and involvement among their subordinates."

Based on this set of paradigms, a participant went a long way towards describing the set of skills that elite schools ideally should inculcate to future leaders.

"I would strive to circumvent students' expectations. And from the moment they would sit in the classroom, I would make it clear that they have entered a space in which the premise is the exact opposite of the conventional proposition that they should simply 'fill their notebooks, and by the end of the course they'll know how to respond to crises.'

I would say: 'You will not be trained to become technical experts—you'll have plenty of time to learn about this stuff, and more to the point you'll have to rely on others who will be more competent than you can ever be in each specific field. But *your* role as leaders will be to restore intelligence, vision, and coherence in environments that will be on the verge of losing all of that.

I would set them to work on simulation exercises: yet not such that they'd be looking for 'the right answers'; I would only select scenarios that did not hold *any* easy answer; and their task rather would be to innovate in order to recover a degree of balance and stability out of chaotic and unscripted situations.

I would tell them to *listen* to others: to practitioners who went through unconventional events. Not however suggesting that these are 'experts' who hold definite answers; but simply that they should listen, and learn from others' insights.

Next, I would have them work on the ground, forming groups that will investigate complex crises, and then report back to their peers on the strategic insights that they drew.

I would also invite specialists of technical fields, firefighters, police; and ask these guest speakers to explain to the class what they will need from future leaders when the time comes: under what set of circumstances they will need decisions, guidance or assets from upper-tier leadership. I would expect firefighters, for instance, to make it clear that they will not ask leaders for advice on 'how to put out a fire': but for critical decisions when disruptions are *'more than just a fire.'*

In a word, I would make it a priority to develop students' strategic ability in the face of unconventional threats: so that it would become the core of their background, of their identity, of their competence.

Lastly, I would tell them: 'You are all together in this; act accordingly. Create a network, keep working with one another, so you can keep learning, keep enriching your experience, across borders and sectors.'"

Towards new criteria for the selection of leaders

There is a clear chasm, of course, between the paradigms that underpin our participants' views, and prevailing criteria that currently determine the selection of leaders. These problematic selection processes take two major forms: they concern both educational patterns, namely the identification of disciplines and intellectual skills by which 'excellence' is measured; and patterns of promotion within organizations, especially at the voting booth in the case of the public sector in democratic polities.

Educational assessment of excellence still suffers from the weight of an antiquated heritage, most notably in certain European countries. Thus a participant called for "new mental frameworks among elite schools, to ensure especially that the selection and promotion of students rely on something other than brilliance in mathematics or physics." Yet the issue lies not only with the promotion of more relevant disciplines among the metrics of academic performance; in a deeper sense, the definition of *what "a beautiful mind" is* needs to shift, and insist upon intellectual creativity, audacity, curiosity, rather than the capacity to learn and regurgitate static bodies of knowledge, with impeccable clarity matched by equally impeccable lack of originality.

Meanwhile, when examining the drivers of promotion and selection within democratic systems, our participants noted with regret that

> "The job description for political candidates certainly varies in each election: but only a fraction of the discussion ever touches upon crisis management skills. And there ought to be more discipline among the public and pundits alike in raising this as an issue in leadership elections, whether at the city level, or county, or state, or national."

Though daunting, the limits of governance in the face of unconventional threats are not set in stone; they can be overcome if leaders are selected based on their capacity to anticipate and respond to these threats. As a participant argued, "so much in response efforts to unconventional crises comes down to leadership, and personality, and relationships. And I think there is a lot that can be done on that front, improving the selection of those who are chosen to play that role in the first place."

A number of colleagues, for instance, highlighted that organizations should strive to circumvent the stun effect caused by unconventional disruptions by recognizing that leaders' personalities can entirely change—for better or worse—under high levels of stress: and therefore by selecting decision-makers based on existing tests that can predict individual reactions in such circumstances. Leaders should be chosen among those who not only hold adequate *knowledge*, based on their past experiences: but who also react well to *lack of knowledge*, in environments characterized by imperfect, confusing information.

"And this plays out differently for everyone; each individual finds his or her own balance between the two."

In the end, "Not everyone can be effective in a crisis cell; organizations need to learn to exclude those who cannot; identify in advance those who do not work well under high stress. And of course this is sensitive work in organizations that have complex turnover." That the task is sensitive should not, however, discourage organizations from taking it on: but simply convince them that they can waste no time to start doing so.

Group dynamics

A danger inherent in any disquisition of leaders' selection processes lies in exclusively focusing on individual skills. A participant helpfully insisted that this was an analytical and strategic mistake.

> "We should not be striving for perfection in one person. Let us not be fooled into thinking that we can somehow turn out the perfect, well-equipped, all-rounded leader! We should not ignore the fact that decisions are made by *groups* of people: and that the *composition* of leadership groups is very important."

The two dimensions, in fact, are inseparable, since tweaking group composition will not help if individuals' culture and skills remain inadequate to confront unconventional events. Yet it is also true that salvation will not come from the emergence of individual, superhuman leaders draped in the cloak of newly redefined excellence, but from the skillful combination of unconventional minds whose inter-personal dynamics are at least as important as their individual qualities.

Conclusion

As we take stock of the road traveled since the launch of our program in 2006, the most valuable result so far certainly is the emergence, coalescence, and maturation of a cross-sector, transatlantic platform for dialogue and innovation. We have successfully turned disparate preexisting networks into a group whose value added has been enhanced, rather than undermined by its eclectic composition; while this variety also replicates, as in a microcosm of crisis response, the complex maps of stakeholders that unusual disruptions bring about.

The present report, held side by side with its 2008 predecessor, amply demonstrates the degree to which our concepts have matured; mechanisms have been tested; and a broad consensus has emerged — all the more powerful for combining approaches whose drivers and underlying objectives remain occasionally different; indeed, thriving on this difference. As a participant put it, "We don't all use the exact same language; nor do we all operate on the same plane. But we don't need to. This is part and parcel of the process: and in fact it reflects our most important paradigm — that if all sides show flexibility and creativity, there is no need for everyone to agree on everything."

Looking ahead, three paths emerge to build upon these dynamics. First, we need to turn from a synthetic effort to create common interpretative frameworks, towards the focused application of our ideas and mechanisms upon specific challenges — in other words, return to "ground level," and to the granularity of our participants' professional concerns, after striving to escape their gravitational pull to lay out a high-plane overview.

This we have endeavored to achieve in 2008-2009, most notably by organizing an *ad hoc* seminar in June 2009 to look back at the A(H1N1) outbreak, examine relevant precedents such as SARS and H5N1, and look ahead at the risks that the new strain could yet pose in the coming months: in the process testing the added value of our ideas and proposals upon the touchstone of this specific threat, and their power of conviction by submitting them to participants who had not contributed to the conversation until then.

Pandemics such as A(H1N1), however, are but one example of looming threats that we know will materialize in the near future. As our proposals aim to effect a culture change that will enable leadership structures to look at unconventional risks with eyes wide open, their ultimate test—and ultimate success—will come from tying together the new vernacular that we have laid out, with a forward-looking endeavor to map upcoming risks: turning from an academic effort that built upon the richness of our participants' past experience, to a policy-relevant drive towards preparing for future contingencies. As a participant noted,

> "We are not yet looking carefully enough at the world *as it will be*, and at the hazards that are coming our direction. We should now combine what we know of future hazards—related to global climate change, global economic change, access to food and water, the use of violence in the international arena—and the mechanisms that we are advocating here for dealing with hypercomplex events. Because we *know* that more of these emerging issues are coming our way."

Lastly, the conversation, and the resulting effort towards reforming leadership culture and organizational structures, must be internationalized. Certainly the Center for Transatlantic Relations at SAIS has been the appropriate setting to start addressing these issues, as Europeans and North Americans share comparable sets of conceptual, political, economic, and societal frameworks, and therefore are the interlocutors most likely to bring about the coalescence of a joint, mutually intelligible agenda. They also remain—for a short time yet—the most powerful stakeholders in responding to unconventional events, and increasingly have become a prime target for this type of disruptions, which they long believed could only affect other, less fortunate parts of the world.

Yet at the dawn of the 21st century, as G8s around us turn into G20s, it would be singularly ironic (and more importantly, counterproductive) to restrict the conversation to transatlantic partners—all the while calling for leaders to broaden their awareness of relevant stakeholders beyond their comfort zone. Specifically relating to unconventional crisis cells, a participant called upon our proposed formats, such as EDF's Rapid Reflection Force, "to open up to different cultures, different mindsets, because crises in our globalized world will compel them to scan the horizon for weak signals across multicultural systems." A colleague most eloquently broadened and summarized the point when he underlined that

> "All of us here live in the same 'Western bubble.' Europeans and North Americans, we represent less than 15 percent of world population! If a disaster affects our interests, but does so outside that bubble, in the Middle East, in Asia, for example—how will we deal with it? How will we interact with local stakeholders? With civil society in China, in India? This will compound problems of 'language' or 'grammar': differences in analytical frameworks, strategic instincts and operational habits. All of us here are familiar with broadly similar Western processes: so we work well with one another; but that's not the hard part."

A crisp and precious description of where we stand at this juncture. So far the going has been easy: now to the hard part.

Annex I: Interviews

The following is a transcript of the short film that was screened in the first session of our seminar (see agenda below). The film was a montage of extracts from interviews conducted by a participant with a series of officials who have lived through unconventional disruptions, and have drawn especially insightful analyses from the experience. It also illustrates the type of pedagogical tools advocated earlier in this report among our recommendations to modify educational practices in leadership courses: as the same participant has screened this and other films with much success in his own classes.

Interview #1: Canadian official

Interviewer — I would like to explore with you for a moment the key problems that characterize emerging crises today: because they have changed since the last century; examine the key issues. And one of these issues is our mental blocks: why are we so reluctant to take into account the new realities, and what can we do to train current leaders, or future leaders in educational institutions?

Canadian official — Well first of all, I think it's very fitting that we recognize that you and I meet on various continents at various times: because that's the world we live in now. The issues that I face in North America are the same issues that you face in Europe. In many instances, because of things like emerging diseases and pandemics, we in fact will fight them together. But we find at events like 9/11 and the tsunami that in fact they involve multiple countries, all at the same time. There were, for example, thirty-five different countries that came to the tsunami.

So I think you're absolutely right: the kind of thinking, the kind of approaches that we need to take to these issues is changing, and we're discovering as we go along that we have to have new approaches. And as you often describe, out-of-the-box thinking has to become the norm, not the exception.

First of all, certainly in speaking to political leaders, and senior people in governments, I always make the point that we will see emergencies, and we will see increasing numbers and increasing severity of emergencies. The debate about whether or not we're having some form of global warming seems to, in fact… —even the die-hard are starting to acknowledge that there are weather effects. And of course the weather effects aren't as obvious as just saying: well, it's hotter, or it's colder. We're seeing droughts in areas where we've never seen droughts. When you see drought, you also see forest fires, for example: we're having forest fire problems like you've never seen, and you see this in Greece, and you see it in California, and you see it in the Yukon in Canada, in arctic areas where we're getting drought as well. And you see heat extreme enough, as you saw in… —and I often talk about the Paris summer [of 2003] and the deaths. I mean, these are catastrophic emergencies.

You see… —unfortunately we all recognize the risk of terrorism; and, you know, we may not have world wars going on, but we have many global conflicts, and we have a very unsettled world right now, and that has consequences.

With travel we see how quickly emerging diseases are going to happen, and we will have a pandemic: the question is, will it be mild, will it be moderate, will it be severe? And we have to anticipate that…, and react accordingly.

We see the effects of things being linked together: whether it's computers being attacked by viruses, and losing the ability… —and computers are obviously controlling huge amounts, ever-increasing amounts of things—or whether it's physical linkage, like our hydro-electric systems. But things can go wrong, either weather-caused, or human-caused, as happened with our blackout.

Interview #2: British official

British official—We should now be beginning to learn that fighting the last war is a waste of time; and that what we need to be able to do is to identify what the real war is now.

The fuel protests that we had in the United Kingdom, where a few hundred people managed to stop the flow of fuel to 27 million vehicles in this country, required us suddenly to understand how fuel was being delivered, from the refineries to the petrol stations; how the minds of the people driving the tankers had been affected by their own industrial conditions: they were reluctant to face the picket lines; the very great passion behind the protesters themselves; and the ability of the public at large to be completely selfish: to ignore the fact that if they simply didn't queue up for petrol, the crisis would not have happened.

Now, we learnt all those things in the three or four days it took to try and get this crisis under control. Nobody had thought about those things before then. The industry had thought about "what happens if we lose supply"; the government had thought about "well, how do we ration petrol if it's short." But nobody had put together social factors, economic factors.... And the systems that run a modern economy.

Interview #3: NYFD official

NYFD official — *In my classes [before 9/11], I always used the World Trade Center as a model of an evacuation. I used it as a model of having a Fire Command Station within the building. It was always a model, model building. None of us on that day expected that building to come down: it was a large fire...* — *and a couple of previous fires that we've had here in the United States, of buildings that have burned for...* — *some buildings apparently as long as nineteen hours, such as in Philadelphia and other buildings in Los Angeles...* — *but we expected the fires eventually to burn out. We knew that we had a lot of people that had died in the crash: we were aware of that. But we never, never once expected that was going to...*

Interviewer — *...So this was completely new...*

Interview #4: New Orleans airport official

Interviewer — *This is somewhat reminiscent of Apollo 13: trying to do the best you can in a strange environment, but you have to save the situation...*

Airport official — *Absolutely; exactly. Apollo 13: a wonderful example of using the lunar module as the lifeboat because the command module was getting steadily colder, and colder, and colder. I mean, a remarkable story, exactly. And it's like that* — *it's: use every resource that you've got, and use it creatively and effectively.*

Interviewer — *And what struck me is that before Katrina, you were [working in] an airport. And suddenly you become [involved in] something else* — *you don't know exactly what it is, but...* — *is it a shelter? is it a morgue? is it a military base? Suddenly you become the first, largest airport in the country...*

Airport official—...*and now it's the largest hospital, the largest emergency ward*—*the largest maternity ward! We had twenty-seven babies born by people who were waiting to evacuate. So: absolutely. That's... the other lesson is that...*—*again, about throwing out the rulebook*—*we have the rulebook for how you run the building and the facility as an airport. We did not have a rulebook for how to run a hospital, or how to run a maternity ward, or how to run a kitchen, or how to run a dormitory... So in each case we had to just talk to all of us and talk through...*—*well, where could we put it, how big should it be, what else is it going to interfere with? And the best example of that was that we put the dormitory for all the relief workers, and the kitchens*—*and most importantly the showers, so they could get clean*—*we put it out where the airplanes normally parked: we used up an area where normally twelve airplanes park, and built this big city. Because it was controllable, it was compact, and it was in the center of the entire airport, so it was convenient for people to get to.*

Interviewer—*So the question is how do I build a city in my airport?*

Airport official—*Right: you just...*—*you do it! And of course, initially, there were people who said: "well, by the book, you should never put this here. It's not appropriate; and it's..." But what it meant was that if we needed those resources, if we needed fifteen people to hop in a truck and go fix something*—*well, they were right there, they weren't..., you know, they weren't a kilometer or two away. They were just right next to our emergency command center, so we could go out and say: "we need folks to go fix this problem." So it was very, very useful to have that resource close.*

And that's...—*probably another great lesson is "close," is "proximity," is "distance." Because you'll lose your cellular phones, your mobile phones; you'll lose your radios, you'll lose your telephones, you will not have the ability to send faxes, email...*—*all of the normal, wonderful things we use to communicate with: you may lose all of them! We lost everything except a few telephones at our worst point: and not our most critical telephones. So communication ends up face-to-face.*

Interviewer—*And one thing that is absolutely essential in order to communicate effectively is to have the same vision of the situation: if some participants want to go by their book, you'll see conflict arise rapidly.*

Airport official—*Absolutely. And all you can do is just remind them that their book doesn't work. And sooner or later, they will learn. But it takes time. And it can be very frustrating. But you have to start...*—*remember: everyone is there to help! But it's true: many of them say, "well, by my book, here is what I should do." And you have to get them just to realize that this is not a normal emergency: and so their normal procedures won't get to the safety and security and life-saving that needs to be done. And so you need to just throw it away.*

Again, another obvious example—*an area where we normally only have commercial passenger airplanes: we had thirty or forty helicopters at a time, giving up their precious cargo. They'd gone into the city, they'd picked people off of roofs, out of attics of houses, out of boats, off of tops of tall trees; brought them to the airport, where they could then get on a regular airplane and get out to safety. And those helicopters were coming in much faster than we could deal with them: so we would have thirty or forty waiting at a time. No one would ever want that circumstance; you know, under* all *the books, you would say: that's not safe, it's not careful, it's much too risky. But we had no choice! We had to get...*—*those people were coming. Those helicopter pilots were going to go, they were going to retrieve those people, they were going to bring them to some place where they could hopefully hand them over to be helped. And in the first day or so, those people were usually in pretty good shape: but by the second, and third, and fourth day, we're talking people who'd been on a roof, in a temperature of thirty or more degrees celsius, for hours, days, no water, no food. These people were in very very bad shape: and of course we had to accept them. And the only way to get them all there was to have a lot of helicopters. But it truly was* completely *not by the book.*

Interview #5: British official, postal services

British official—*I think probably a point which is worth emphasizing is just how confusing, messy, difficult this [the anthrax crisis] was, and how little we knew. Because this wasn't the kind of crisis where there is a clear focus. There was no explosion, there was no flood, there was no fire: it very subtly, over a period of weeks, emerged that there was a major problem, as the material literally seeped through the United States postal system. It's not a disease where people are immediately affected: there is an incubation period; people were presenting with symptoms over a long period. We in the United Kingdom, or in Europe, had no idea whether this was a United States phe-*

nomenon... — in fact no one's actually been arrested for the crime, so we still don't know exactly what the origin was. It was only a couple of weeks after 9/11, so there was an obvious connection with al-Qaeda — I don't believe it's true, but that was an assumption one could not dismiss at that stage. And there was a great deal of lack of understanding of the nature of the problem: what was happening in the United States — they did magnificently in trying to disseminate information through the postal world, but initially of course they just didn't know themselves what was going on. And I think above all, it was a threat outside the experience of all postal managers. Postal managers, at least in the U.K., grow up with the threat of a letter bomb: how to deal with it, how to deal with a suspicious item, is ingrained, is imbedded... people do the right thing because of long training and long instinct. This was entirely outside of our experience.

Interview #6: New Orleans bank official

Interviewee *— As I drove, I kept dialing into these conference calls. While I made my way across the state of Louisiana and eastern Texas, the news got worse and worse from New Orleans, as more and more levees were breached, and more and more water entered the city. And as that happened, the telecommunications network of BellSouth began to fail — massively fail. And at the end of the count, some thirty-one central offices were totally put out of commission. It's an unprecedented occurrence. [An official at] BellSouth told me that in his fifteen years in the company he'd only known one central office to fail catastrophically, completely. And here they were: thirty-one stations out.*

So essentially, the whole of southeastern Louisiana and southern Mississippi was without communications: no voice or datalines. And our whole network, including our backup network's strategy was really dependent upon our branches and computer center in New Orleans being connectable. Although we may have been driving it from a computer in Chicago, and from a network control center in Houston, we depended on the physical infrastructure of the network throughout South-East Louisiana and Greater New Orleans.

Interview #7: British official

British official *— I think the one... — if I had one priority, it would be to make people think about networks. We live in a society that's constructed of networks, at local, regional, national, and transnational level.*

To distort Newton's theorem — Newton said that for every action, there is an equal and opposite reaction — I think in the modern world, for every action, there are multiple reactions, across the networks. And every action that one takes, particularly in a crisis, or in preparing for it, or thinking about it, one should be thinking about the effect on all *the people who might be involved. There needs to be an analysis of the stakeholders who have a stake in these things; and of what might be disrupted.*

People need to build *time… — crises rob us of time; the thing that we can train people to do at university is to think about how they build time into the consideration of these things. One way is in preparation, in understanding how networks are built, and therefore being able to map them very quickly in a crisis; and secondly, during the crisis, to build time for decision-makers by assembling those maps accurately and quickly, and putting them in front of the decision maker. That gives the decision-maker time to make proper decisions.* Rhythm *gives him or her time to make proper decisions. Without that time, and without that appreciation of networks, I think we're probably lost.*

Interview #8: French official

Interviewer — For a long time you were among the top officials at [a French elite school]; if you still held that job, in this or another educational institution, and you thought about the type of leaders that you wished you could train, that you needed now:… what are your views regarding how best to prepare students not merely to "answer the multiple-choice question properly," or write good academic papers, but to meet this type of challenge which are becoming increasingly prevalent?

French official — When I would rank my students, the grading system was rather narrow; getting the top grade was a rarity. I would only give it to students who I believed were unconventional leaders; those who, in addition to their remarkable knowledge, ability, and character, weren't content with following the way that was laid out for them, but could set off on their own path, and take others with them — be it through their strength of mind, their charisma, or their desire to challenge the status quo. And to those only I would grant the top grade, when I thought them capable of playing that role.

I still would have the same approach today. But I think that I would speak differently about the challenges that await them once they leave the school. At the time, I thought that all they would encounter was administrative routine, conformism, so they could do just fine if simply driven by the will to excel, rather than to lead. Today, though... —mind you, I always insisted that the world was a dangerous place. Because it seems to me that elites draw their legitimacy from confronting danger; otherwise, there is no reason for them to exist. But today I would be much more stern in describing the challenges that they will have to meet out there. Because I think it's a tough, tough world. It's a world that has lost its bearings—nobody has a sense of direction any longer; and those entrusted with high responsibilities must prepare to fulfill them in this world that has lost its balance.

Yet I would change nothing on... —skills which I thought crucial at the time are still paramount—except that our curriculum did not prepare students for this type of situations—and I am not sure does so any better today. So I would speak to them in a very direct, very precise, very sobering way about risks. The first thing I would tell them, I think, would be this one certainty we have, that we have no idea what shape risks will take! As we confront new crises everyday: literally everyday something new emerges.

Annex II: Participants

Pierre Béroux
  Chief Risk Officer,
  Electricité de France

Richard Bissell
  Department of Emergency
  Health Services, University
  of Maryland — Baltimore
  County

John Bridges
  Executive Director, National
  Preparedness and Homeland
  Security, USPS

Esther Brimmer
  Deputy Director, Center for
  Transatlantic Relations, SAIS

Drew Bumbak
  Director, Center for
  Emergency Education and
  Disaster Research,
  University of Maryland —
  Baltimore County

Nan Buzard
  Senior Director, Interna-
  tional Disaster Response,
  American Red Cross

William Dab
  Professor, Centre National
  des Arts et Métiers, France

François-Xavier Desjars
  Director, Crisis Management,
  Société Générale

Jacques Drucker
  Counselor for Health
  Affairs, Embassy of France
  in the U.S.

Stephen Flynn
  Senior Fellow for National
  Security Studies, Council on
  Foreign Relations

Rune Froseth
  Chief of the Strategic
  Planning Unit, OCHA, UN

Xavier Graff
  Chief Risk Officer, Corporate
  Risk Department, Accor

Mike Granatt
  Partner, Luther Pendragon,
  U.K.

Xavier Guilhou
  CEO, XAG Conseil, France

Malachy Hargadon
  Environment Counselor,
  Delegation of the EU
  Commission in the U.S.

Mike Hickey
  Vice President, Government
  Affairs & National Security
  Policy, Verizon

Deane Johanis
  Manager, Emergency
  Planning, Greater Toronto
  Airports Authority

Patrick Lagadec
Director of Research,
Ecole Polytechnique, France

William Lyerly
Special Assistant for Global
Health Security, DHS

William Malfara
Director, Response Staff
Deployment, American
Red Cross

Janice Maragakis
Vice President, Corporate
Communications,
Accor (North America)

Russell Miles
Tsunami Program Manager,
Humanitarian Response
Department, Oxfam America

Robert Noonan
Managing Director, Business
Continuity, Société Générale
Americas

Alexis Pierce
Office of International
Affairs, DHS

Rob Quartel
CEO and Chairman,
FreightDesk Technologies

Gilles Rhéaume
Vice President, Public Policy,
Conference Board Canada

Anne Richard
Vice President, Government
Relations, International
Rescue Committee

Larry Sampler
Deputy Coordinator, S/CRS,
State Department

James Schear
Director of Research,
National Defense University

Christian Sommade
Executive Director, European
Homeland Security
Association

Larry Steffes
Vice President and Assistant
General Counsel, Veolia
Transportation

Mike Theilmann
Senior Liaison Officer
from Public Safety Canada
to DHS

Benjamin Thibault
Homeland Security Program,
French American Foundation/
France

Tjip Walker
Warning & Analysis, Conflict
Management & Mitigation,
USAID

James Young
Former Special Adviser to
the Deputy Minister, Public
Safety Canada

Annex III: Seminar Program, April 10–11, 2008

Thursday, April 10

9:00 a.m.–9:15 a.m. **Welcome Addresses**

9:15 a.m.–10:15 a.m. **Session 1—Unconventional Leadership: Reforming Crisis-Management Cells**
Leadership: Pierre Béroux (EDF)
To frame the spirit and purpose of the debate, Pierre Béroux will present strategic lessons resulting from unconventional crises or simulation exercises that Electricité de France has recently confronted. A short film will also be screened with interviews of especially insightful leaders outlining their strategic analysis of recent unconventional events.

10:30 a.m.–12:30 p.m. **Session 2—The Challenges of the "Unthinkable": Early Warning, Culture, and Hypercomplex Disruptions**
Based on the framework laid out by Session 1, this will be a round-table presentation of our participants. Each will be given three minutes to describe their own vision of strategic challenges raised by unconventional events, and their analysis of unanticipated pitfalls, innovative tools for action, and promising proposals for reform—rather than describing at length the facts of a specific crisis, which in many cases will already be familiar to our participants. As a basic guideline, we propose that these short interventions be framed by the following questions:

1. What was the **essence of the unconventional crisis** in question, and did it prove difficult to identify as such in an appropriate or timely way?

2. What were the **critical pitfalls** to avoid, and had they been properly flagged ahead of time? If not, how did you identify them?

3. **Who were the stakeholders**, and did they differ from your traditional partners in planning and response efforts? How did you go about making sense of such confusing "maps of actors," and

rebuilt working coalitions?

4. In the course of confronting the crisis, were **unconventional initiatives** taken, such as enabled your organization to change the dynamics of the event to its advantage? If so, what were they, and what were the intellectual/leadership frameworks and processes that elicited and enabled them?

2:00 p.m.–4:30 p.m. **Exercise 1—Confronting Simultaneous and Insidious Disruptions**
Leadership: Pierre Béroux (EDF), Mike Granatt (Luther Pendragon), Patrick Lagadec (Ecole Polytechnique).
In keeping with the spirit of our initial simulation exercise in March 2007, we will not produce a pre-set scenario aiming simply to test participants' familiarity with a preordained plan. The aim of this exercise will be to familiarize them with unconventional operational or strategic approaches developed by our session leaders: namely EDF's Rapid Reflection Forces in a French context, and Mike Granatt's "hubwatch" concept in the U.K.
Participants will be divided into several working groups, assuming the roles of:
1. Unconventional crisis cells

2. Red teams, "working on behalf of the crisis" and adding unanticipated disruption into the scenario at critical moments

3. Political leaders (sub-national, national & international institutions)

4. The "outside world": victims, greater public, unusual stakeholders, old and new media, and third countries.

Based on the scenario of recent crises confronted by our session leaders, but with significant input from all other participants as appropriate, we will aim to emphasize and develop unconventional analytical approaches, operational mechanisms, and strategic outlooks.

4:45 p.m.–5:15 p.m. **Presentation**—The European Union and Unconventional Crises: Political Dynamics and Operational Mechanisms
Malachy Hargadon—Environment Counselor, Delegation of the EU Commission in the United States

7:00 p.m.–8:30 p.m. **Reception** at the Residence of France's Ambassador to the United States

Keynote Speech: **Stephen Flynn** — Senior Fellow for National Security Studies, Council on Foreign Relations. Author, *America the Vulnerable* and *The Edge of Disaster*.

Friday, April 11

9:00 a.m.–11:00 a.m. **Session 3 — A "New Social Compact": Redrawing Cross-Sector Allocations of Tasks** (the Case of the Pandemic)
Leadership: William Dab (Conservatoire National des Arts et Métiers, France), Jim Young (formerly Public Safety Canada), Mike Hickey (Verizon)
Three experts with backgrounds respectively in a national government, private sector multinationals, and international public health organizations will be asked to frame the debate by sharing their views on the most challenging issues involved in cross-sector, international coordination in the face of cross-border, societal threats such as a pandemic.

11:20 a.m.–1:00 p.m. **Session 4 — The Way Forward**
Our participants will be divided into three working groups examining three topics with the aim to develop policy recommendations. Consistent with the avenues for reform highlighted in our initial seminar and the resulting report, the topics addressed will be:
A. Enhancing Systemic Resiliency

   Leadership: Mike Hickey (Verizon), Robert Noonan (Société Générale)
B. Complex Maps of Actors: Ensuring the "Alignment" of International Responders

   Leadership: Jim Young (formerly Public Safety Canada), Rune Froseth (OCHA)
C. A Generational Challenge: Education, Knowledge, and the Culture of Leaders

   Leadership: Richard Bissell (University of Maryland & FEMA Emergency Management Institute), Patrick Lagadec (Ecole Polytechnique)

1:20 p.m. – 3:30 p.m. **Exercise 2 — The Problem with Plans and Pre-paredness Standards: Improving Processes and Outcomes**
Leadership: Mike Hickey (Verizon), Anne Richard (International Rescue Committee), Jim Young (formerly Public Safety Canada).

Our participants will be divided into working groups, each combining "public," "private," and "humanitarian sector" representatives (though participants from one sector will be encouraged to "assume the identity" of a different sector in order to see the issues from an unconventional standpoint).

Based on the scenario of crises confronted by our session leaders, but with input from all other participants as appropriate, these working groups will each be asked to develop the skeleton of a plan, but more importantly to explore effective inter-sector and trans-national planning *processes*, to tackle three main issues highlighted in 2007 and summarized in the subsequent report: i.e.

1. How to see the loss of critical resources and infrastructure as a founding paradigm of our plans, rather than an "unthinkable" obstacle, in order to ensure that workable systems can be rebuilt in spite of such disruptions;

2. How to develop international, cross-sector databases of available resources to improve the coordination of complex response efforts;

3. How to create allocations of critical strategic or civic responsibility ahead of a crisis (or more broadly, "social compacts"), to ensure that each sector or country states clearly in advance what responsibility it is willing to take on when an unconventional crisis hits.

Session leaders will advise the working groups based on their expertise of their own sector, and finally will chair a plenary discussion based on a comparative overview of the planning outlines, and more importantly planning dynamics, developed by all working groups.

Annex IV: Contents of 2008 Report

Unconventional Crises, Unconventional Responses: Reforming Leadership in the Age of Catastrophic Crises and Hypercomplexity (Washington, D.C.: Center for Transatlantic Relations, 2007)

Introduction
The Need for Inter-Sector and International Dialogue
Reforming Traditional "Crisis Management"
The Project

A Survey of Unconventional Crises
Catastrophic Events
Insidious Events
Cascading Events
Hypercomplex Events

Lessons Observed
The "Liquefaction" of Systemic Foundations
The Crucial Role of Information and Knowledge
The Importance and Ambiguities of Leadership
The Challenges of Inter-Sector Coordination

The Way Forward
Building Response Mechanisms Into "Normal" Systems
A New Social Contract: Redrawing Inter-Sector Allocations of Tasks
From "Behavioral" to Resource-Based Planning
Unconventional Leadership and Response: "Rapid Reflection Force"
Reforming the Culture of Leadership: A Generational Challenge

Conclusion: Phase II

About the Author

Dr. Erwan Lagadec is a SAIS Foreign Policy Institute Fellow at the Center for Transatlantic Relations. He also teaches at the Fletcher School of Law and Diplomacy at Tufts University, and the Elliott School of International Affairs at The George Washington University. His work focuses on transatlantic issues in homeland security, European civilization and politics, and U.S.-EU-NATO relations. A French national, Dr. Lagadec holds a D.Phil. in history from the University of Oxford (2004). In 2007-8 he was an affiliate at MIT's Security Studies Program. In 2005-6 he was a postdoctoral fellow at Harvard University, and remains affiliated with its Center for European Studies. In 2004-5 he was a Public Policy Scholar at the Woodrow Wilson Center and a Visiting Scholar at SAIS, looking back at French-U.S. relations during the 2003 Iraq crisis.

A Reserve Officer in the French Navy specialized in international relations and policy planning since 2005, he has worked as an outside consultant for the French Foreign Ministry's Policy Planning Staff (2003, 2005); the Delegation for Strategic Affairs at the French Ministry of Defense (2005); the U.S. mission to the EU (2006); the military mission at the French Permanent Representation to the EU (2007); and the military mission at the French Embassy in the United States (2008).

The first report of Dr. Lagadec's ongoing project at SAIS, *Unconventional Crises, Unconventional Responses: Reforming Leadership in the Age of Catastrophic Crises and Hypercomplexity*, was published in 2008. Dr. Lagadec co-authored a 2006 report for Electricité de France (EDF) and the French Navy's Chief of Staff that analyzed the response of Gulf Coast critical infrastructure providers in the wake of Hurricane Katrina; he also co-produced a 2005 report on "The Rehabilitation of Civilian Ports in Crisis Situations" for the Delegation for Strategic Affairs at the French Ministry of Defense.

About the Center for Transatlantic Relations

The Paul H. Nitze **School of Advanced International Studies** (SAIS) is one of America's leading graduate schools devoted to the study of international relations. It is based at Johns Hopkins University, one of the nation's premier research universities. Further information is available at http://sais-jhu.edu.

The SAIS **Center for Transatlantic Relations** is a non-profit research center that engages opinion leaders on contemporary challenges facing Europe and North America. The goal of the Center is to strengthen and reorient transatlantic relations to the dynamics of a globalizing world. More information can be found at http://transatlantic.sais-jhu.edu. The Center serves as the coordinator for the American Consortium on European Union Studies (ACES), which is a partnership among five national-capital area universities — American, George Mason, George Washington, Georgetown and Johns Hopkins — to improve understanding of the European Union and U.S.-EU relations. The Consortium has been recognized by the European Commission as the EU Center of Excellence in Washington D.C. CTR also contributed to the creation of the Congressional Caucus on the European Union, and remains closely associated with it. In 2009 the Center was named by *Foreign Policy* magazine as one of the "Top 30 Go-To Global Think Tanks." The Center leads international research activities of the Johns Hopkins-led National Center for the Study of Preparedness and Catastrophic Event Response (PACER), named as one of the five U.S. National Centers of Excellence in Homeland Security by the U.S. Department of Homeland Security. This group comprises seventeen different university institutes across the United States, and studies a range of homeland security challenges.

In 2005 the Center organized and hosted the event *Atlantic Storm*, based on the scenario of a simultaneous biological terrorist attack in Europe and the United States, which included high-profile participants such as Bernard Kouchner and Madeleine Albright. In addition, the Center has published extensively on homeland security issues, e.g. *Transforming Homeland Security: U.S. and European Approaches*; *Transat-*

lantic Homeland Security? Protecting Society in the Age of Catastrophic Terrorism; *Protecting the Homeland: European Approaches to Societal Security — Implications for the United States*; *Terrorism and International Security*; *Fighting Terrorist Financing: Transatlantic Cooperation and International Institutions*; *Role Reversal: Offers of Help from Other Countries in Response to Hurricane Katrina*; and *Five Dimensions of Homeland and International Security.*